From Humble Beginnings...

Writing your first book appears to be much like establishing credit for the first time. With no previous writings in my portfolio, and not being a celebrity or recognized authority on my chosen subject; I automatically became a "bad risk" to all publishing houses.

Against these odds, this book was written, edited, typeset, composed, copyrighted and printed. With the talented resources and encouragement of my immediate family it has been a rewarding experience.

The contents of the following pages were written for you. Karen and I trust you will gain something from the sharing of our personal cancer story.

Other books by R.G. Rockman, Jr.:
None.

Credits:
None.

Reviews:
None.

Testimonial:
I beat cancer. It's now a part of the past. Our past.

Published by
R.G. ROCKMAN PUBLICATIONS
1537 N. Leroy St. —Unit F
Fenton, Michigan 48430

First printing, May 1991
Revised edition, May 1992
Revised edition, August 1994

Printed in the United States of America:
Thomson-Shore Printing, Inc.
7300 West Joy Road
Dexter, Michigan 48130

Typeset and composition by Dean C. Ouellette.

Cover design by Deborah A. Rockman.

Distributed by R.G. Rockman Publications.

Rainbow Man

Richard G. Rockman, Jr.

FOREWORD

During my yearlong battle with cancer many of life's lessons were indelibly imprinted within my mind. Of those many lessons, quite a few left just as large an impression on my heart and soul. The end result was that these learned lessons were assimilated into my personality. Good or bad, most of them are there to stay. Hopefully, most of these fall into the good category.

I beat cancer and I believe many other human beings can also defeat this dreaded disease. We all have the capability, the only thing some of us lack is the knowledge and real commitment. The voyage through disease to a healthy body is long and difficult but it's worth the effort because that effort can mean the difference between life and death...health and sickness. It was not an easy journey for me and will not be for other cancer victims. But the truth is that if I can do it — so can you!

Rainbow Man is a guided tour through the world of cancer. The journey is full of unscheduled stops and unmapped routes. That's okay. Don't let it get you down. Remember, at one time I was also a rookie on this uncharted course. I am now cancer free and a walking, talking picture of health. At the end of the road, the same rainbow I found can be waiting for you. It's an all encompassing rainbow of good health with your place safely designated beneath its prismatic arches. You won't need a camera or sack lunch for this tour; an open mind and the desire to be rid of terminal disease are all that is required.

The circumstances which unfold en route to our destination of a cancer free body are essential. Sometimes they are depressing, sometimes they are humorous, always they are necessary. These uncontrollable events establish the credibility of my experience. They emphasize the fact that I am just like anyone else faced with the threat of cancer...scared and vulnerable. Without the credibility of these events my story would just be an overstated opinion. My goal is to share my personal experience and let the reader draw his or her own conclusions.

If you enjoy happy endings then I invite you to take a journey with me down cancer lane. A journey down a darkened street that will force even the strongest of us to face our ultimate loves, fears and emotions. Those of you who know me personally will know me a little better; those of you who don't know me at all, will at the least know me a little. To know me is to know what I discovered. To know me is to know that **CANCER CAN BE BEATEN.** To know me is to have HOPE against cancer and FAITH in the final outcome. Follow me through circumstances and situations that were out of my control but part of my life. Come with me and discover why you treat cancer with medicine but beat cancer with God.

> **For God has not given us a spirit of fear;**
> **but of power, and of love, and of a sound mind.**
> *2nd TIMOTHY 1:7*

INTRODUCTION

We live in a whirlwind world. Although it frustrates me, I admit to being an unwilling participant. The dizzying pace of the 20th century amazes me on a daily basis. The schedules and "must do" events that dominate our lives are overwhelming. The avalanche of electronic communication equipment that interrupts and distracts our attention hour by hour is overpowering. Radios, VCR's, TV's, recorders, computers and finally, telephones all contribute to a normal day of 20th century confusion.

Some of us accept this pace as a fact of life. Some of us resent the pace but don't know how to slow it down. Some of us even love it and wouldn't want it any other way. ALL OF US are affected by it every day of our lives.

Without a doubt, this 20th century lifestyle had held me captive for quite a few years. I resented my daily participation and yet, realized that each succeeding month and year it seemed to get worse. I had less time for family and self and spent more time frantically working and functioning at the world's hectic pace. I was a husband first; a dad second; and the family breadwinner third. The trouble was that third place got most of my attention and time. When I did get home from work, very often there was not much left of me to give to the first and second place in my life.

The habit-forming pace which had controlled my life for many years came to a sudden halt on February 11, 1989. This was the date I entered the hospital with what appeared to be severe "flu" symptoms. Two days later I was diagnosed with cancer. It wasn't just cancer, it was a BIG cancer.

On February 13, 1989 a large, malignant tumor was discovered in my lower right abdomen. The tumor also enveloped the base of my spinal cord. This was the day I had to answer the biggest question of my life...how do I deal with cancer? More to the point, how do I handle the roller coaster of emotions that this dreaded word — *cancer* — brings with it? A roller coaster with many more dips and curves than highpoints. I kept asking myself. How can I make sane, rational decisions when my knowledge is so limited concerning this monster called cancer? Why do I feel so out of control even though the few options available are mine to exercise? I want to make good decisions and choices but where and when do the decisions and choices stop? Last, but certainly not least, how could a merciful God allow this to happen to me? I may not be a saint but I'm basically a good human being, aren't I? This MUST be a mistake.

Often, the events and circumstances did not seem real. It's as if they were happening to someone else and I was just an omniscient observer. The world seemed like it was operating in full gear all around me but was meshing without me. My life felt like it was "on hold" as people and events churned through their normal daily routine all about me. I felt totally isolated; completely alone and motionless. It was as if I was watching the world through a one-way mirror. Then reality would settle back in, usually escorted by tumor induced pain, and I would know once again that I was indeed the cancer victim and another life or death decision beckoned. What doctor...what hospital... what treatment? Decisions, decisions and more decisions, accompanied by mind-boggling questions. Would radiation halt the growth of my cancer? Would chemotherapy kill my tumor? Would the cancerous cells spread to other parts of my body? Would my wife and our kids be alright as I went through treatment and surgery? Would I even be alive after treatment and surgery? Was I really just a statistic, a plus or minus on some doctor's survival chart?

These are some of the haunting, black thoughts and mind messages I struggled with each and every hour. The unconscious demand to make new decisions seldom let up. It was a fatiguing, depressing and demoralizing routine.

All these emotions are very real for the cancer victim. They are a stark reminder of how utterly lost and helpless the cancer patient feels during moments of his or her own ordeal. These feelings accent the fact that cancer is not just a physical battle, it is also an emotional battle. My confirmed belief is that the cancer victim must confront cancer on the emotional level in order to defeat cancer on the physical level. This conclusion is drawn from personal experience and I trust, insight. It has been gathered through my own long hospital stay; coexisting with other patients; and through volunteer work. I don't claim to be an expert but I do claim to be keenly observant and quietly sensitive to other cancer patients' situations.

If I didn't feel I had something positive to offer I would never have attempted this story. I would leave the next cancer victims to their own resources and go on with my own life and business. The problem is that I have an intrinsic nature that basically likes most people. Not really a problem, more like a dilemma of heart and conscience.

The heartfelt conclusion I've come to is that I want to offer other cancer victims a shortcut to what I discovered. I want to offer them hope and impress upon the latest victim the belief that cancer is a storm which can be overcome! The cancer patient can choose to fight and strive to live. There can be a rainbow on your horizon at the end of this ravaging storm.

With the American Medical Association projecting that within 10 years one out of every four Americans will be affected by cancer during their lifetime, I feel humbly compelled to offer anything I possibly can. One out of every four Americans means a lot of sons and daughters; moms and dads; and even grandmas and grandpas will be struck with this terrible disease. As the medical profession searches daily for new cures and treatments, the cancer patient must help him or herself by battling with everything they have at their disposal. And that begins with his or her own attitude. Set your attitude in line with a higher authority. Very simply, when your back's against the wall and you're searching every avenue of escape, put your faith in a God which none of us on planet earth have ever met. The unseen God which masterfully created and designed the human body. Put your hope in the peace and health that *He* offers through his words in the Bible.

In conjunction with any remedy you may utilize, from chemotherapy and radiation to cobalt implants and experimental drugs, don't lose contact with that "higher authority." Give God and your medical doctors something to work with...get attitude TOUGH. Admit that this situation is out of your control. Reach for the peace of mind that only God and *His word* can give as you attempt to maintain a successful fighting attitude. Meet cancer on your terms and with all the ammunition you can bring to the fight. YOU CAN WIN with a will to live and God as the last word.

How do I know that accepting a God we've never seen is the route to real peace of mind? That's easy...because I looked everywhere else for that inner peace. I was left to contemplate God because modern medicine considered my original diagnosis to be terminal. Specifically, three doctors looked at me as if I was already dead. They spoke to me about survival statistics and then they talked to me as if I were just that — a statistic. In their mind, a soon-to-be dead one. The major design of writing this book is to help someone else who is facing now, or will in the future, what I already faced — life threatening disease. My secondary motivation is to let the world know that I am more than just a statistic — I'm a flesh and blood human being. And a very much alive one at that!

My story is written out of purpose, not necessity. The world could have gotten along just fine without my opinion on cancer or any other terminal disease.

But, the world is not who I am writing this for; I'm writing it for the individuals who don't know what they're up against when cancer suddenly strikes. The ones who don't realize that cancer must be confronted emotionally BEFORE it can be defeated physically. I'm writing it for the human beings who will try to go it alone fighting cancer. Relying only on themselves. I'm writing it for the human beings who hand their cancer to the doctor by unconsciously saying, "I'm in your hands, doc' — cure me." I'm writing it for the human beings who are so completely lost and scared that they give up and wait around for cancer to claim them through death. Most importantly, I'm writing it for the human beings who don't know there is a compassionate God, much less believe in him as a source of healing.

This book is directed at all of you. Before you turn another page, understand something right now. Cancer is extremely personal. It is your fight and no one else's. All the help and support the world has to offer cannot alter the fact that it is YOUR life hanging in the balance. If you choose to take cancer on all alone, you most likely will lose. If you put the sole responsibility of your cure on your doctor's shoulders, he most likely will fail. If the words "you have cancer" scare you into total submission, you will most likely die. Finally, if you neglect to ask for God's help, you will undoubtedly be meeting cancer on its own deadly, emotional terms. Forgetting God would be a short-sighted mistake. Because after mankind's medicine has been exhausted, God may be the ONLY hope you have left.

Understand something else; there is no compromise with cancer, either you beat it or *it* eventually beats you.

DEDICATION

To my wife, Karen Marie, and our five children; Melissa, Cheryl, Ricky, Stacey and Randy who fought cancer right alongside me. Your personal battles and sacrifices did not go unnoticed. Your love and devotion tipped the scales of life and death in our favor. You made the difference.

Contents

Chapter 1

CANCER STRIKES

It's time to introduce myself. My name is Richard Glenn Rockman, Jr. I live in a small Midwest city in southern lower Michigan. My wife's name is Karen [or my pet name K.M. which stands for Karen Marie] and we've been married for over 19 years. We have five beautiful children, three girls and two boys, ranging in age from 10-18 years old. The girls are Melissa, Cheryl and Stacey; the boys are Ricky and Randy. This is Karen and the kids' story as well as mine. They also coped with change, insecurity, doubt and rumors on a daily basis. Cancer interrupted their lives every bit as much as it did mine.

My saga actually begins with my brother. It was December 15, 1988 and I recall quite vividly that it was a cold, blustery, overcast day. A typical late Fall afternoon for Michigan, threatening to snow with the sky's dark clouds gathered in foreboding clumps but not quite down to the freezing mark yet. Craig walked into my office, pulled up the chair across from my desk and sat down for a heart to heart talk. The door swung closed as I looked from the window behind my desk to his face — I could instantly see worry written all over it.

We had worked side by side for the last ten years and handled many job related problems with this similar beginning. Not overly concerned, I asked, "What's going on brother?" He propped his feet up on my desk and proceeded to tell me he had just come from the doctor's office. "While I was taking a shower last night I noticed that one of my testicles was hard, like an egg. So first thing this morning I made an appointment. They scheduled me for an ultra sound test tomorrow." Craig paused as our eyes met, "Rick, Dr. Hamilton told me it could be cancer."

Dazed, I stupidly said, "Cancer!...You're kidding!" Seated at my desk, with that dumbfounded look on my face, memories flashed through my mind of all the business decisions we had made in the past sitting here just like this. They all seemed terribly insignificant now. I tried to be nonchalant and talk positive until the test results were in but my words were probably as hollow sounding as the inside of my stomach felt. I was now very concerned.

In September 1988, just four months earlier, we had sold all three businesses to a group of investors from Mt.Clemens, Michigan. The three (3) businesses were compatible parts of our father's newspaper, a bi-weekly publication named *Tri-County News*. While we were still discussing that terminal word "cancer" there was a knock on my office door. It was one of the new owners. He came in and asked how things were going. My brother has a dry humor and in typical fashion he made light of the situation by replying in a squeaky, high-pitched voice, "Just fine, Jerry." Excluding Jerry from our prior cancer conversation, Craig and I both laughed. By alluding to the possibility that he could be running around with one less testicle in the near future Craig's facetious comment had taken the edge off the situation. For now, humor had the last word.

The humor was gone by 3:00 p.m. the next afternoon. Craig got a call from Dr. Hamilton's office confirming everyone's worst apprehensions....it was a cancerous tumor. He handled the shock remarkably well as he left the office and went home to inform Beth, his wife, and decide on their course of action. As Craig shared later, you can never really prepare for bad news of this degree. "You think you can but you can't. It's like a flood hits you and you're drowning and swimming...all at the same time."

This was not my first introduction to the disease of cancer but Craig's diagnosis was really hitting close to home. Then, and even more so now, we had a close brother relationship. We were tight. Since he was almost two years younger, it really made me agonize for him as I tried to understand what he was going through.

In 1977, my dad lost his second oldest brother to cancer. That was a traumatic experience for the whole family, watching Raymond die at 37 years old. His death was a real tragedy as it left four young children fatherless; yet I wasn't as close to the situation, or Raymond, as I was with Craig. A striking parallel existed in that Craig had just turned 37 years old [November 1988]. This ironic fact added a rather chilling effect to the whole situation.

Another brush with cancer occurred in March of 1985. Our family had to deal with this cancer scare when physicians in Florida thought my then 55 year old father had *Brights disease*, a severe kidney disorder. These same physicians also discovered "spots" on his liver and kidney during a routine C.A.T. scan, which they thought to be cancerous.

After nearly submitting to very serious surgery in a Southern Florida hospital, dad came back to Michigan for another opinion. This was at the urging of a specialist who I recalled had saved one of my best friend's mother's legs from bone cancer back in 1978. This doctor went against the consensus medical opinion and opted for experimental procedures. He was willing to combine delicate surgery with radical radiation treatments versus the proposed amputation. The technique was successful and my friend's mom fully recovered.

The name of this specialist was Dr. James Cox. Through my friend's wife [she and Dr. Cox are first cousins] I was able to contact him and ask what he would suggest in my dad's situation. He advised on a second opinion from University of Michigan Hospital in Ann Arbor. Thank God, dad listened. Following weeks of sophisticated tests his kidney disorder turned out to be high blood pressure [hypertension] and sugar problems from borderline diabetes. Also, the Michigan doctors found no *spots*, otherwise known as tumors, on my dad's liver or anywhere else. The liberal expertise of Dr. James Cox would soon be called on again...in my brother's behalf.

For Craig, events happened very quickly. He was referred to a doctor in Mt. Clemens and this doctor suggested surgery immediately. By Monday, December 19, 1988 Craig was in surgery and having the malignant tumor removed. On December 21st the hospital released him with orders to take it very easy; he was home by 10:00 a.m. that morning. My wife, Karen, met me at work and we drove over to see Craig and Beth to give them some moral support. Unbeknownst to Karen, it was also a trip to answer a couple of nagging questions on my mind.

When we got there they were both sitting on the sofa in their new room addition. It radiated warmth and hospitality as the sun shone through the large, tiered windows positioned overhead and on the south wall. Construction had just been completed on this "great room." The richly colored decor seemed to belie Craig's recent surgery and confrontation with cancer. Resting comfortably, he looked excellent considering the five inch incision he was nursing from the operation. The only noticeable effects were his slow and stiff body movements. At that time, the doctor's felt they had "got it all" and the prognosis was for no follow-up treatment. Craig's form of testicular cancer was diagnosed as seminoma and the chances for complete recovery fell into the 90 percentile bracket. He and Beth looked relieved and relaxed as they shared this information.

All of us were talking about the family Christmas party coming up on Friday which Craig and Beth still insisted on hosting. Eventually, Karen and Beth headed for the kitchen to raid some of the Christmas goodies. Their departure gave Craig and me a chance to talk privately. I asked him if there was anything he was keeping from us that the doctors had mentioned. Confidently he said, "No, I've told you everything the doctors have told us and you know I'll level with you if any curveballs are thrown at me."

That reply was good enough for me so I turned the talk in my direction. With no hesitation I blurted out what had been gnawing at my mind for days, "I've had pain in my groin area for quite awhile now...should I be checking myself for lumps, bruises, bleeding or what?" I pulled my pants down and pointed to where it seemed like I always had a knot and sometimes pain-filled pressure.

Trying to compare notes I asked, "Is this where you had

pain before the tumor showed up?" He shook his head sideways in the negative as I added, "It hurts mostly when I'm driving or sitting."

Craig reassured me that he'd had no symptoms or pain in that area so it was probably nothing to worry about. In fact, he reminded me that the only pain I ever mentioned in the past was in my back and that the "knot" in my groin was probably a muscle pull or at worst, a hernia.

We let it drop and I recall feeling guilty about even bringing up "my pains" after what Craig had just been through. The doctors had suggested very strongly to Craig that all the males in our family have a complete physical in the near future due to the type of cancer found in him. As he was emphasizing this point the girls walked back down into the great room and we let all cancer conversation cease. After all, it was Christmas 1988 and we had much to celebrate and be thankful for...especially Craig's cure!

The entire family did get together that Friday and we thanked God for our many blessings. Again, Craig's good fortune foremost on all our minds. We posed for a family portrait that day which included grandparents, parents, children and grandchildren. Altogether there were twenty-two of us; in other words, the whole Richard Rockman, Sr. clan.

Like most holiday seasons it was a very busy time and even busier with my youngest sister slated to get married on December 30th. Lisa and Rick [yes, another Rick in the family — we already had four — and we were running out of nicknames] were married in the Linden Presbyterian Church and the reception was held in our home.

It was a beautiful ceremony but the date and festivities stick out in my mind for other reasons. Friday, December 30, 1988 was the same day that I received a complete physical and clean bill of health from my doctor. Aware of my brother Craig's problems, the doctor had scheduled me for an ultra sound on January 4, 1989 at a Flint radiology clinic. "Just to be safe" were his cautious words. By Friday, January 6th the Doctor's office had called and confirmed that the ultra sound test was clean. To me, this was a green light which emphatically implied that any pain I'd been having was apparently no cause for alarm. I didn't know it at the time but this was just the beginning of some ugly ironies headed our way. My "good checkups" would soon come back to haunt us.

Chapter 2

MY TURN
[And Craig's Again]

On January 12, 1989 Craig got a call from his doctor stating that the x-rays and C.A.T. scan he underwent following surgery indicated some small tumors in his lymph node system. C.A.T. is an abbreviation for Computerized Axial Tomography. This is an elaborate diagnostic machine which scans the human body in cross-section views.

Armed with this new information, the doctors scheduled a lymphangiogram to pinpoint the exact location of the tumors and decide on what treatment they would propose. I distinctly remember that this test was no fun for my brother because the dye is injected under local anesthesia. Medically speaking, a lymphangiogram is a long, impressive name for a lymph node test where a small incision is made across the instep of both feet and dye is shot up through the patient's arteries. The dye is monitored as it travels through the arteries and past the lymph nodes; small, compact structures of tissue which lay in clusters along the network of arteries which travel up and down the human body. Diagnostically, the test is designed to locate and highlight any malignant masses within the lymph gland system.

This sudden turn of events took the whole family by surprise. We were naive about the disease of cancer to say the least. Although Craig's newly discovered tumors may have enlightened us all concerning the gravity of cancer, it certainly did nothing to cheer us up. I was struggling through an aerobics class when I got a call at the studio from Karen telling me about this latest batch of bad news. This particular night left a deep impression on my mind. When I hung up the phone from Karen I suddenly realized that cancer is not something that you just treat and forget. Cancer did not appear to let go of its victims graciously or entirely, and that bothered me! It felt as if someone had just knocked the wind out of me. I wondered how Craig was handling this latest development.

Once again we contacted Dr. James Cox. This time it was to ask if he would give a second opinion on the recommended follow-up treatment by Craig's doctors. With more than just professional courtesy he replied, "Certainly, send the reports to me in Houston as soon as you receive them." With his casual manner and confident attitude it was reassuring to touch base with Dr. Cox.

As we all worried about Craig, life went on. For me, that meant working 70-100 hours a week. My own work ethics and a demanding, competitive typesetting business dominated most of my waking hours. Even though we had sold our respective businesses in the package deal I mentioned in *Chapter One*, Craig and I had agreed to stay on board until December 31, 1989. We hoped to help ease the new owners into the newspapers' established business climate. The smooth transition we were aiming for kept me working just as hard and long as I did when I owned the business. In fact, in some instances I worked harder because I did not want any loose ends when ready to move on next December. My dad, Craig and I continued to put in a lot of time at the office.

The newspaper represented 31 years of labor for our father and 10 years apiece for Craig and myself. As our father's brainchild, *Tri-County News* was started in 1957 on a song and a prayer and had been nurtured into a thriving $1.5 million a year business. Although Craig and I had grown up working off and on at the family run "Tri-County" we did not officially come on board until 1978. From the very beginning it was a rewarding challenge for all concerned. We considered every employee of *Tri-County News* a true asset and tried to treat them accordingly. This attitude promoted loyalty and enthusiasm. The concept is what made me, personally, work so hard. I learned a long time ago that it is much easier to lead by example than strictly by orders. From top to bottom, everyone produced and carried their own weight. At the top, health problems were about to strike again.

On January 21, 1989 the fatigue of long hours and stress of newspaper deadlines caught up with me. Following a night of high fever and severe lower back pain, Karen took me into the Flint Osteopathic Hospital [FOH] emergency room. Our family physician was out of town for the weekend. It was Saturday and I sure didn't want to spend hours sitting in a hospital ER, but if I wanted relief the wait was a must. An intern got to us in less than an hour. We discussed my symptoms and by then the fever had leveled off at 102 degrees. I recall telling the young intern that my back hurt at the base of the spine and had for quite a few months. I told him that I had not been able to sleep on my stomach for the last few months and that it seemed like my lower back always hurt more when I went to bed. He did some probing and prodding and treated me for a low grade kidney infection. On the way home, we filled two prescriptions and from there I went into work. After all, tomorrow [January 22nd] was Super Bowl Sunday and I certainly didn't want to miss the celebration of this annual football extravaganza. Sure enough, by Sunday the fever was gone and I was feeling fine. Or so I thought...

Three short weeks later, on February 11, 1989 I was back in the very same hospital, sitting in the very same emergency room, with the [you guessed it] very same symptoms. The only thing missing was the very same intern. Apparently, he had the weekend off. As before, no real warning preceded the seemingly instant sickness that gripped me. Just the day before, Karen and I had taken her parents into Detroit for a day of fun and entertainment. We spent the whole afternoon roaming the display floor of the 1989 Boat Show [held at Cobo Hall in downtown Detroit] and we spent the evening at the Fox Theatre watching the Broadway reproduction of *South Pacific*. Everyone had a great time, although my back hurt me more than usual as we sat through the theatre performance. Karen said I complained about my back all night...I remember mentioning it a couple of times. It must be marriage that allows two unlike perceptions of the same circumstance. Oh well, Karen was probably right in her assessment. It SEEMED like I complained only a couple of times.

The routine was repeated that we went through on January 21, 1989. I had the same high fever, back pain and now, sweaty clamminess was added to the list of symptoms. The doctors talked kidney infection again but I had no blood in my urine so they ruled that and possible kidney stones out. After about three hours in the emergency room the doctor on duty spoke to my family doctor and they decided to admit me for observation. By then the fever had subsided; the backache had let up; and the clamminess was gone. Once again, the symptoms were slowly fading but the cause was beginning to bother me. Under duress, I consented to admission for observation.

Sunday morning arrived with me in a semi-private room on the 3rd floor at Flint Osteopathic Hospital. The nurses took more blood samples and I was scheduled for a battery of x-rays covering the chest, back and lower abdomen sometime before noon. I wanted to leave and go home because I felt okay now. The symptoms had mysteriously disappeared again. Karen quieted me down and convinced me that we still needed to find out what was causing the high fever and sweatiness. The blood work and x-ray results came back which were taken in the morning and reflected that nothing conclusive had turned up. Prompt for his morning rounds, our family physician, Dr. Hamilton, ducked into our room and told us that I could go home but warily added, "I'm not completely satisfied with the negative test results." The hospital's on duty resident doctor was prepared to discharge me but Dr. Hamilton reminded us that this was the second time in three weeks that I'd experienced the onset of these very same symptoms. He insistently suggested, "You're here already, Rick, let's try a couple more tests and see if we can find out what the real problem is." A C.A.T. scan was ordered for 7:00 a.m. Monday.

It was still Sunday, late in the afternoon. Karen and I were just small talking as an FOH surgeon and intern entered our room. Dr. Hamilton had asked the surgeon to take a look at me and do an exam of my abdomen and lower back. Politely,

Dr. Slaubaugh introduced herself and the intern accompanying her on rounds. Without delay she began her examination by asking me several questions and softly pressing in my lower abdomen area. As she was pushing a silent alarm went off in my head. For the very first time I felt that something was drastically wrong down there...I could feel slight pain and much pressure in the right side of my abdomen. She was gentle in her probing and upbeat in her bedside manner but she "clucked" a couple of times as she completed the exam. Turning to the intern, Dr. Slaubaugh offered an opinion as she returned her hand to my lower right side, "I think I might feel something in this area." He took a turn inspecting my abdomen but couldn't seem to feel anything. They asked what tests were scheduled for tomorrow. I told them a C.A.T. scan was ordered and they seemed to agree with that as they headed for the door. With a wave, Dr. Slaubaugh said she'd see me tomorrow and wished us goodnight.

The alarm that sounded earlier was now on hold. I consciously refused to think about the panic which I'd felt for a few seconds when the surgeon was probing with her fingers. Karen stayed awhile longer and then went home to get the kids ready for school in the morning. Negative thoughts were pulsing to the tip of my brain but I still wouldn't let myself say, or even think, cancer. As I wrestled with these thoughts I tried to relax and get some much needed sleep. Logic won out over anxiety and I finally convinced myself once more that it couldn't be anything serious. The last effort I recall was rolling over onto my stomach to sleep and the pain in my lower back forcing me onto my side in the fetal position. It was the same dull, pressure pain I'd had for months. The next thing I knew a nurse was saying, "Good morning, they're here to take you for the C.A.T. scan, Mr. Rockman."

When I got to the diagnostic test area an old high school friend came out to say hello and tell me he'd be conducting the C.A.T. procedure. Gary is the chief diagnostic technician for the scanner and has been doing it for years. The test took about 25-30 minutes. From there, I was taken to a waiting area before being escorted back to my hospital room. A short time later, this is where Gary found me sitting. Awkwardly, he said, "Rick, you have a tumor." He began to inform me of the large mass the C.A.T. scan had just located in my lower right abdomen and back. He confided that they weren't sure if it was a benign or malignant growth but the consensus was towards cancer. The majority opinion was leaning towards malignancy because of its size, shape and location. As I was sitting there absorbing the shock of *CANCER* possibly being *IN MY BODY* the same surgeon who had examined me the night before approached.

Dr. Slaubaugh had a sympathetic smile for me as she quickly said that they would like to do a needle biopsy on the tumor to let pathology confirm whether it was benign or malignant. I cut her off before she could say anymore and told her point blank that if it was malignant, chemotherapy was not an option I would consider. She looked at me as if I had just pronounced my own death sentence and somberly asked, "Why, Richard?" I related how I had watched my uncle die 12 years earlier of stomach cancer. "My opinion, then and now, is that the chemotherapy did as much to kill him as the cancer. I made up my mind back then that if I ever faced cancer it would be without chemotherapy." Choosing her words carefully she said, "Why don't we discuss this after the biopsy results are back. You do not have to decide anything right now." I responded with complete finality, "There is no discussion as far as I'm concerned."

That's the way we left it as an orderly wheeled me back to my room. By then it was about 7:30 a.m. but all I could think of was telling Karen. She usually came up to the hospital around 8:30 or 9:00 in the morning and I sure didn't want to give her news like this over the phone. Impatiently, I waited for her arrival. In my own mind, I came to the realization that the tumor was going to be malignant and that this was turning into a very bad daydream. I remembered the pain from the night before. As I looked out my 3rd floor window, a thousand disconnected thoughts were trying to storm my brain at the same time. While still waiting for Karen I took 3 or 4 phone calls from relatives and friends and maintained the facade of, "The doctors don't know anything yet. We'll let you know when they do." Karen had to be informed before anyone else. My sincere wishes were that I didn't have to tell *anyone* that I had this thing called cancer growing inside me. The knowledge made me feel tainted and vulnerable.

It was almost 10:00 a.m. when Karen came in like she always did; with a big smile on her face. This reminded me of the main reason I was attracted to her 20 years ago — she was such a natural human being at loving and caring. She could see beauty where there was none. I let her tell me about running errands and getting the kids off to school before I broke the news. Her spontaneous response was, "It can't be!" This was more an emotional reaction to the news than a flat denial of the facts. From there she wrapped herself in my arms and hugged me very tight as she whispered, "Let's wait and see. Let's just wait and see."

We agreed on consenting to the needle biopsy exam. I shared with Karen the panic I had felt the night before as the surgeon was probing my lower midsection. Neither one of us are what you might call "crepe hangers" but I did want to prepare K.M. for the worst as my fear from the night before was still very fresh in my mind. It felt like all the clocks were on "hold" as I recalled the two hours spent waiting for Karen to get to the hospital that morning. Seemed like the longest two hours of my life but we would soon learn that we had many more hours of apprehensive waiting in store for us. Like a fair weather friend, I started saying prayers to a God I had pretty much ignored the last few years. Obviously, God didn't know this was Rick Rockman, Jr. and that I refused to have cancer. I prayed anyway.

Before long, FOH orderlies took me down to the C.A.T. scan room again, this time on a surgical stretcher to prepare for the needle biopsy. This is a test where the doctor freezes the suspected tumor site with novocaine injections. Then, sample tissue is acquired from the suspected internal organ or mass. After my lower abdomen was numbed with four or five shots, the doctor proceeded to insert a long, hollow needle into the tumor area as the procedure was monitored by the C.A.T. scan operator. This was to make sure no vital organs were inadvertently pierced while extracting a sample of the tumor tissue. The pathology department would make the final determination on whether the specimen was malignant or benign. The doctors wanted to know and I HAD TO KNOW for my own benefit. No one had to persuade me the procedure was necessary in my case. Likewise, no one had to remind me that the needle in my stomach was not a pleasant experience. Within an hour I was back once more in my room and waiting for the pathology report. More waiting, more tense anxiety and more apprehension.

Around 3:30 p.m. that afternoon the preliminary pathology report came back and confirmed the tumor was malignant. Karen and I were prepared for this moment but it still left the same hollow feeling in my stomach that I'd felt for Craig. Some tears slipped down Karen's cheek as she fought hard to hold her emotions back. Her eyes momentarily flickered with fear and doubt, then she quickly recovered. Later, she confided that it felt as if someone had grabbed ahold of her heart and tried to wrench it from her body upon hearing the report's finding. From the earliest moments my wife's strength was evident. Before this saga was finished I would be truly amazed at her reservoir of emotional strength.

Monday, February 13, 1989 was winding down for us when our family physician once more came by on his daily rounds to tell us he was aware of the biopsy results but not to give up hope. He said the chief oncologist and surgeon would be in to see us tomorrow. For lack of a better name, I considered the oncologist a tumor technician. Karen was well aware of my feelings concerning chemotherapy treatment but rather than argue she handled me with her usual finesse and let the issue drop with, "Let's wait and see what the doctors say."

We did not sit around moping. That night we briefly phoned our relatives and closest friends to let them know what we were up against. Quite naturally, they were all rather stunned. Especially, since we had all just gone through this kind of news with my brother Craig. After a few more "must make" phone calls, Karen and I discussed how we would present my cancer diagnosis to the kids and then she went home to do just that. I called the house and asked all the kids to be home when mom got there because she had something to tell them. It was difficult not to pass on the bad news over the phone but Karen and I agreed that the best way was in person. We knew they would have a thousand questions and fears.

Around 10:00 p.m. I called home again to make sure Karen's talk with the kids had went alright. Considering the circumstances and the kids' capacity to comprehend the threat of cancer, it went as well as it could. All alone, with just the hospital quiet to keep me company, I recall thinking, "So much for the tests and good checkups I had six short weeks ago." There was no bitterness, no resentment, and no finger pointing; only bewilderment. The irony of the circumstances leading to the discovery of this large tumor in my abdomen seemed to consume my thoughts. Unfortunately for me, early detection had been missed six weeks ago. Now, in addition to my younger brother, I was fighting cancer. I went to sleep that night swearing that cancer was not going to claim me as a victim.

Another day and more bad news. My type of cancer had been diagnosed as sarcoma. This meant very little to me at the time because I was under the impression that cancer was cancer. Sometimes, ignorance will take you a long way in certain situations; Tuesday, February 14, 1989 was one of those times. I was soon to discover that all cancers are NOT the same. Some types are considered more treatable than others. It appeared that I had one of "the others." Naively, I'd already made up my mind that "I" was going to beat cancer...just hadn't figured out exactly how yet.

My mind was travelling faster than the speed of sound as random thoughts tumbled rapid fire through my brain that winter morning. *This was just a bad rap — something I had to go through and get finished. Let's see...I'd verbally, and mentally, ruled out any form of chemotherapy, so...just have to be tough and bull my way through this cancer thing. With chemo ruled out the only other treatments I'd heard of were cobalt and radiation. That fits perfectly into 'my' plans because Dr. Cox is a radiation expert. Maybe I should say some prayers...no, I don't have time to pray; have to get ahold of Dr. Cox again. Hmmmm, the last time was for Craig. We're going to wear this guy out with our family's cancer problems. Need to see if he will take me as a patient, or better yet, refer me to someone in Michigan who treats cancer with radiation. Should be able to get back to work in a couple of weeks, hope they can manage things until then. Karen will be there for the kids, she can handle them alone until I get out of here. I'll call home every night.*

As you can see, I had this cancer thing all figured out. This was just like any other problem or challenge I'd come up against over the years; you meet the problem head on and it takes care of itself. I was definitely up to the challenge and would beat it faster and better than anyone. Man, did I have a lot to learn about cancer!

My first lesson was about to begin. The head of the Flint Osteopathic Hospital Oncology Department dropped into our room about 2:00 p.m. that Tuesday afternoon. Oncology is the branch of medicine which treats tumors, so Dr. "B" was certainly in the right place, considering the malignant mass recently discovered inside me. I had just climbed back into the hospital bed after taking a long corridor walk which enabled Karen and her mother to share some private time together. Helen had come down from East Tawas, Michigan the night before to give her daughter some moral support and help us with the kids at home. Her presence was a steadying influence for Karen. I was daydreaming and the ladies were chatting about nothing in particular as the chief oncologist strode into our room and introduced himself.

His attitude was polite, his stature was dignified and his manner was direct. Promptly, Dr. "B" got down to business. He stated that I had a very big tumor in my lower abdomen. Described as larger than one of my hands, it was touching my spine and pinching the vena cava and possibly aorta that ran along my spine. He explained that the vena cava and aorta were the large veins that return blood flow and supply circulation to the lower extremities. If I understood correctly, the aorta pumps the blood down and the vena cava is the pipeline back. Kind of like a North/South expressway of large veins which run along the spine. His diagnosis was sarcoma in the fourth stage. The prognosis was that most patients with this specific cancer, and in this stage, live less than 90 days. He concluded the prognosis by stating that modern medicine had experienced very little success in the treatment of this particular tumor. His recommendation was immediate exploratory surgery to remove the tumor and spleen, then take sample tissue of my other vital organs as they attempted "to get it all." He had me tentatively scheduled for surgery at 8:00 a.m. the next day. I thanked him for his time and said we'd give him an answer on the surgery as soon as possible.

Well, my first cancer lesson was finished and I wasn't too thrilled about the lesson plan. Remarkably, we all quietly controlled our teeming emotions until the doctor left the room. Following his departure a few moments of hushed silence ensued. I broke the quiet when I turned to Karen and said, "I don't care what they call this thing in me...we'll beat it." My words weren't enough. Tears began to cloud her blinking eyes as she fought their uncontrollable release. Softly, I repeated, "It'll be alright K.M....it'll be alright." From there I went out in the hallway to attempt to give all this morbid news some sort of perspective. This left Karen with her mom so they could talk and console each other.

Alone, with just my thoughts, I walked the hospital corridor. I realized for the first time that this monster inside my body called cancer was trying to consume me from the inside out. It made me feel terribly dirty and contaminated to have that "thing" growing inside me. It was an ugly, scary feeling.

Our minister happened to drop in for a visit shortly after the head oncologist had departed. Don's visit was a Godsend, especially for Karen. I'm sure he didn't realize that ten minutes ago we had heard my carefully worded death sentence as he spread some love and kind words. His encouragement gave Karen the strength she needed to get through that afternoon.

Don left us — but not before he had reassured Karen that the decisions we were about to make would be confirmed in her heart and she need not worry about doing right or wrong. He convinced her she would "feel" what was intrinsically right and God would put it in her heart.

Soon after Don left, Karen and I decided we wanted a second medical opinion. When Dr. "B" had given us his diagnosis and started mentioning biopsies, exploratories and spleen removals, I had mentally noted that a second opinion would make me feel much more comfortable concerning any future decisions. As much as I wanted this filthy tumor removed from my body the notion of a second opinion just seemed to feel right. Karen had been talking Houston, Texas and Dr. Cox for the last day and a half anyway. Logic suggested that maybe our doctor in Texas could refer us to a reputable cancer specialist closer to home. Especially, if he couldn't examine me personally. Comfortable with our choice of action, I tried to contact Dr. James Cox at his office.

Within two short hours, Dr. Cox's personal secretary returned our initial phone call and informed us that Dr. Cox was fulfilling an out of state speaking engagement. She kindly gave us a number to try and reach him in Bethesda, Maryland. We missed him at his hotel when we phoned but he called us back at the hospital between train rides to his next lecture commitment. He didn't hesitate when I told him our situation. He offered to admit us to his resident hospital, M.D. Anderson Cancer Clinic in Houston, Texas as soon as we could get there. We had made up our minds that if Jim offered we were going down there for a second opinion at the very least. We told him "thanks" and immediately started making arrangements to fly to Houston. The first step in those arrangements was to cancel my impending surgery at Flint Osteopathic Hospital. By choice, the exploratory surgery scheduled by Dr. "B" would be missing the main character — me.

Although we had always wanted to see Texas, I don't think sightseeing was on either of our minds as we began to make preparations to go out west. The kids were our primary concern. Their welfare and ability to cope were our number one priority.

We waited for Dr. Hamilton to come by on his hospital rounds that evening and told him of our decision. He was very gracious and helped get the ball rolling in gathering all of my medical records and test results from his office and FOH. All the records which we requested to take with us to Houston would be ready by Thursday afternoon and I was being discharged the next morning, which was Wednesday, February 15, 1989.

We would soon be heading for the *Lone Star State* and a second opinion on my verbal death sentence delivered at FOH.

Chapter 3

TESTS, TESTS and MORE TESTS

At 7:35 a.m. on Friday, February 17, 1989 we were on a Northwest Airlines jet and headed for Hobby Airport in Houston, Texas. Karen's mom had volunteered to stay with the kids so we had one less burden on our minds. Neither of us knew what to expect when we got to Houston. We did know this was going to be a fight to the finish.

After a bumpy flight into Houston we found a cab and had the driver take us into the Medical Center complex where M. D. Anderson was located. And what a complex it was! About 8-10 square blocks of nothing but hospitals, research centers, and medical colleges. Quite impressive and at the same time quite staggering. I remember thinking, *There must be a lot of sickness around if all these hospitals and support centers are needed.* The observation proved to be accurate. There was a lot of sickness out there and much of that sickness was a tenacious monster called cancer. We had been referred to the Mayfair Hotel by Dr. James Cox's office so we went directly to it and reserved a room. The Mayfair was right across the street from M.D. Anderson Cancer Clinic. By mid afternoon we were in Dr. Cox's office asking about the admitting procedure. Dr. Cox was absent so we settled for making arrangements to be admitted on Monday, February 20, 1989 at 8:00 a.m. From there we went back to our hotel and camped by the phone anticipating a long weekend of anxious waiting.

Patience is NOT one of my virtues. Karen handles that department because she is patient enough for both of us. When Monday morning finally arrived I was chomping at the bit to get started. Naively, I was still under the impression that this cancer in my body was a problem that could be taken care of in a few short weeks. I'd already mentally rejected the "less than ninety days to live" prognosis delivered back at FOH in Michigan. I just wanted the doctors out here to operate, give me the radiation zaps and I'd handle it from there. Again, I seemed to have it all figured out. Karen subtly [maybe more sarcastically than subtly] reminded me that if I was going to be my own doctor, why had we flown so far to get a second opinion. As usual, she was right.

There were many other patients being admitted that morning so we sat and waited our turn. The more I scrutinized the faces of other patients and visitors scurrying about the premises of M.D. Anderson, the more I realized that people were coming to this facility from around the world as well as from across the United States. This realization was both impressive and at the same time gloomy. People were evidently opting for treatment here because of its excellent reputation. At the same time, it was depressing that SO MANY PEOPLE needed cancer treatment. After a couple of hours, I was admitted on an out-patient basis for testing. From admissions we were directed to the records station to receive a schedule for the next five days of testing I would be undergoing. The only test scheduled for that Monday was to have blood drawn at the infusion therapy station. I went to the blood station after leaving the records department and had my first of many, many blood samples drawn at M.D. Anderson.

On the preceding Friday we had been told that Dr. Cox, under his new title as Vice-President of Patient Affairs, would be back in his office on Monday. Both of us wanted to meet this man who had touched our lives on three different occasions and concerning three different cancer problems — meaning my dad's, my brother's and now mine. Prodded by curiosity and gratefulness, we asked for directions to a pre-arranged 1st floor waiting room in the Lutheran building of M.D. Anderson. This building housed some administrative offices but was primarily the hospital wing used for in-patient treatment within the complex. Dr. Cox was supposed to be at that location. Karen and I must have looked as lost as we felt wandering the maze of hallways, offices and medical stations because when we asked for directions a friendly hospital employee volunteered to escort us to the area.

Upon arriving, we were informed that Dr. Cox was in a meeting and that he would see us in a few minutes. Shortly thereafter, I spotted a man garbed in the traditional white medical robe coming directly towards us. Karen nudged my arm and we both knew this distinguished looking gentleman had to be Dr. James Cox. We stood and formally introduced ourselves. At the same time, we thanked him again for working us into his busy schedule. He struck me the same in person as he had in talking long distance over the phone. His approach was one of genuine concern. He radiated conservative confidence and his progressive, upbeat attitude was contagious. Karen and I felt easily comfortable in his presence. We both liked him immediately. He informed us that he had looked over the x-rays and records we brought with us but didn't want to conjecture. "Let's wait for all of Rick's tests to come back and then we'll sit down and assess the situation," Dr. Cox suggested. We left his office buoyed by the feeling that my cancer dilemma was going to be in good hands. Also, it was nice to finally be able to put a face with a name and voice.

The next three days consisted of testing, testing, and more testing. Our days were spent at the hospital undergoing blood tests, x-rays, needle biopsy, ultra sounds, C.A.T. scans, etc. Our nights were spent trying to occupy ourselves constructively.

One of the highlights of our evenings was to call home and touch base with the kids. Even though we knew very little concrete information at this point, we tried to keep the kids and rest of our family informed. Craig and Beth called us at the hotel on Wednesday, February 22nd. They wanted to know how we were doing and tell us Craig had taken his second radiation treatment that morning at University of Michigan Hospital in Ann Arbor. Craig concluded the long distance call by telling us he had felt no side effects yet from the radiation treatments. That was good news because we spent a lot of energy worrying about them and I know they fretted over us constantly. I think Craig was more worried about my welfare than he was concerned about himself and the aspects of his own cancer. As I mentioned earlier, we were close. Even though his prognosis was better than mine, Karen and I never lost sight of the fact that he was also battling cancer. They were in our thoughts and prayers daily.

M.D. Anderson was huge and unfamiliar to us so we were assigned a hospital "tour guide." Our guide was officially called a patient coordinator; to us, she was a genuine Texas sweetheart. Her kind direction was greatly appreciated as she happily escorted us to the location of each test. This was another impressive fact concerning the M.D. Anderson facility, they actually had an auxiliary staff to assist showing lost (new) patients their way around the hospital. The first few days at M.D. Anderson we certainly fit into the "lost patient" category. It was a twelve-story collection of hospital rooms, labs and offices. The clinic and surrounding complex were overwhelming.

About now, you may be wondering what happened to all the original test records we brought with us from Michigan. I know I was wondering why I had to take many of the same tests over again at M.D. Anderson. The answer was simple. The new tests were taken for comparison against the old ones and to gauge any new developments in the tumor. Once again, Karen reminded me..."That's what we are here for...a second opinion."

Friday, February 24th rolled in and I was scheduled for an early morning spirometry test [i.e. a lung capacity determination] and then consultation with a surgeon. We ended up seeing two surgeons that Friday. Neither discussion would later be classified as a pleasant experience. Both surgeons were still under the diagnostic impression that I had sarcoma in the fourth stage of development. With that supposed knowledge my future looked pretty bleak in their estimation. The pathology report from my second needle biopsy exam and some other test results were still incomplete at this time.

We saw Dr. "A" a little before noon. Outside, the sun was shining and the temperature was a mild 60 degrees. These are great weather stats for the month of February to born and raised Michiganders. Inside, the atmosphere was a different story. The surgeons were about to send an ominous cloud of doom our way. Karen and I were apprehensive but really didn't suspect the confirmation waiting for us. We trudged up to the second floor and had a seat in the waiting room.

After a long wait, my name was called and we were ushered into one of the examination rooms. Dr. "A" came in 10-15 minutes later. My first impression was that his physical stature made him look more like a middle-aged marathoner than a surgeon. He was kind of tall, lean and tanned. Introducing himself, he quickly told us that he may not be able to handle our case because he was leaving for a skiing vacation the next day. He shared with us what he knew from the test results that were back. Carefully, he explained that the exams I'd underwent had narrowed the tumor species down to the probability of either lymphoma or sarcoma. Of these two types of tumors, he said that lymphoma was medically considered the most treatable. He stated emphatically, "There is no good type of cancer — but sarcoma is a 'big, bad devil' to deal with." We listened quietly.

Following his explanation and a few moments of silence I said what was really on my mind, "Dr. 'A' I just want you to cut this piece of crap out of me, I feel completely contaminated by this thing." Surveying our faces, he replied in an understanding voice, "We can do that, and I'll get everything I can while we've got you on the operating table, but there are no guarantees that you get all of the cancer cells in surgery." Soon after this exchange, Dr. "A" politely excused himself and left the room. He returned shortly to tell us that his peer, Dr. "W", was going to see us in case we opted to do surgery before he returned from his planned vacation. Up to the fourth floor we went — to meet with Doctor "W".

The reception area was crowded with patients when we arrived at Dr. "W's" clinic station. Eventually, we were ushered into another examination room. In the solitude of that little exam room Karen and I discussed having surgery in Houston. Karen was not convinced that surgery was the best course of action. Conversely, I was convinced it was the ONLY course of action. Dr. "W" entered the room and our talk abruptly ended. It was time to listen again. Drawing another first impression, I decided Dr. "W" looked like a misplaced college professor. He appeared uneasy as his eyes probed us through thick, brown, horn-rimmed bifocals and over a neatly trimmed mustache. While he introduced himself in a soft-spoken, articulate voice our eyes met just long eniugh to get the distinct feeling he was measuring our capacity for bad news. Continuing to visually compare him to his surgeon counterpart, I shifted my body to lay back tentatively on the exam table.

After completing a brief physical examination of my abdomen he leaned up against the wall by the door. In a reserved manner he told us that *"you have a big, ugly cancer inside your lower abdomen, Mr. Rockman."* I thought to myself...*these guys really get descriptive when talking about cancer...and these two consultations are not exactly making my day.*

It soon got worse!

Dr. "W" proceeded to tell us in no uncertain terms that their inclination was towards sarcoma in identifying the tumor. He continued by saying, "In your advanced stage the prognosis does not look real good. The problem with sarcoma is that no matter how many times we surgically remove the tumor growth, it seems to come back in the general vicinity of the primary site and stronger, more resistant than before." I interrupted at this point by asking, "Can't you use radiation to shrink it or at least stop the growth?" He hesitated for a moment like he was debating how to answer my question. Then, in a restrained tone, he explained, "Both chemotherapy and radiation have been relatively ineffective in medically treating this kind of tumor. The survival rate, Mr. Rockman, is less than 10 percent."

Karen was seated at the side of the examination table and behind me. Being a nurse herself, she knew exactly what a "less than 10 percent" survival rate implied. As I looked over at her following Dr. "W's" pronouncement, I could see her slump, like all the air had gone out of her body. She started sobbing softly. Dr. "W" saw that she was upset and graciously excused himself. I let him get completely out of the room. After the door closed, I stepped down from the exam table and went to Karen as her sobbing turned to hysteria. I held her in my arms and tried to console her by stating in as strong a voice as I could muster, "Let them think what they want, this is not going to beat us and I am not going to give in to cancer. I promise." She sobbed harder as I continued to hold her.

These were uncontrollable tears, the culmination of almost two straight weeks of agonizing news. She seemed to need to release the pent up emotions inside her more than the tears themselves. As Karen struggled to regain her composure we waited for the doctor to return, each of us quietly taking refuge in our own thoughts.

The words I had spoken to Karen were still echoing through my mind. Truthfully, I wasn't anywhere near as positive about my fate as the strong words I had conveyed to her tried to indicate. Over and over, I repeated to myself, *"This cancer is not going to beat me."* Before my cancer struggle was finished I would use this method of verbal commitment again and again. Inside I was battling fear and doubt while outside I was calm and collected. It was a contradiction of terms and attitudes but I felt if I said something enough times, gradually, it would become a part of me. I needed the inner conviction that my mental repetitions seemed to temporarily afford. It was a lot of false bravado; but it was right for me and my situation. This approach would pull me through some very tough days and nights in the not-so-distant future.

We were still awaiting the return of Dr. "W" when a nurse came in and told us, "Your consulting doctor will contact you as soon as possible, you can get dressed and leave now." She asked us to stop at the desk on our way out and take our medical records back to patient routing. I knew we would have the whole weekend ahead of us and I didn't want this cloud of doom hanging over us until the following Monday. I took Karen's arm and decided to head straight for Dr. Cox's office on the first floor.

Aloud, I hoped that he was in and would be able to give us a minute or two of his time. We desperately needed to hear his reassuring expertise. Jim came right out from his interior office and I'm quite sure he could tell by the look on Karen's face that something was definitely wrong. The words *Sar-*

coma, survival rates, lymphoma, and less than 10 percent rolled out of our mouths before Jim held up his hand and cut us off. He calmly related that the pathology report was not confirmed and that they were still leaning towards the possibility of a rare form of testicular cancer for diagnosis. His words were like a soothing ointment. They didn't promise anything specific but they did present hope and temporary relief. Jim took it a step further, with a quick phone call he set it up for us to see M.D. Anderson's chief oncologist that afternoon. He insisted we would like this gentleman and convinced us the consultation would be to our benefit. We thanked Jim for easing our minds and headed to station #17 where Dr. Logothetis, head of the Genitourinary Oncology department, was located. Desiring anything which resembled good news, we wanted to keep this unscheduled appointment.

The waiting area at station #17 was also terribly crowded with patients but the meeting ended up being well worth the delay we endured. Dr. Christopher J. Logothetis bestowed upon us the first real positive words we had heard concerning my cancer plight since the tumor was discovered on February 13th. He was convinced that I had a rare form of testicular cancer called mixed-cell non-seminoma in the fourth stage. He persuasively stated that it could be treated and that there was a good chance of complete recovery. The ONLY negative thing he said was that I had to undergo chemotherapy to combat this type of cancer. By the time we left his conference room he understood this was a big stumbling block for me.

First impression means a lot. Especially under these circumstances. Dr. Logothetis' knowledge and understanding of cancer, and its treatment, were immediately obvious. So were his powers of persuasion and diplomacy. His quiet confidence fed our hopes. We asked if he would take me as a patient. His answer was a quick, "Yes." With solemn appraisal, he explained what our obligation would entail. "You have to commit the next six months of your life to nothing but beating this cancer, Richard. You cannot worry about your wife, your children, your work, or any financial difficulties... Can you do that?" he asked.

I thought for a moment as he looked directly at me then

replied, "Yeah, if I have to I can do that. But, I just don't know if I can submit to chemotherapy. I don't believe in it as medicine and I don't have faith in the results." He politely let me finish as I asked point-blank, "Why can't you just cut this hunk of junk out of me...it makes me feel like my insides are contaminated with nuclear radiation."

My one track mind was exposing itself again. This was the second or third time TODAY that I had asked this question. I just couldn't seem to grasp that this cancer battle was NOT going to be waged on my terms or conditions. Some of us are slow learners.

Dr. Logothetis took a deep breath as he chose his words carefully. "You're used to giving orders and pretty much controlling your own environment, aren't you, Mr. Rockman?" I had no idea where he was headed with this kind of statement but I answered honestly, "Yes, pretty much."

He seemed to study me as he stated categorically, "We used to do things your way, Richard. In fact, only a few short years ago, your type of cancer was considered absolutely terminal. We took patients in your same condition to surgery, did the best we could cutting away all the cancer and then told them 'we think we got it all' as we sent them home to recuperate. All of those patients are dead now." There was a pause as he let this ill-fated disclosure sink in. "We [the medical profession] found out the hard way that microscopic cancer was almost always left behind. Weeks, months, and even years later, cancer would reoccur in those patients and it was usually too late to help them. That's why we no longer advise doing surgery first. If at all possible, we try to shrink and kill the tumors with chemotherapy and radiation before we operate."

Logothetis continued to eye me, reading my face and wondering if his declaration of facts had hit home. He finished his lecture by adamantly declaring, "The statistics support treatment with radiation and especially chemotherapy BEFORE surgery. If we're going to have a chance to cure you, Richard, you need to allow us to use the tools we have proven can work. In your case that is chemotherapy."

With reservations I reluctantly bent to the persuasive

powers of Dr. Logothetis and the common sense instincts of Karen. I had the unfortunate impression that Dr. Logothetis was being generous in his optimistic appraisal. But, with all the negative reports earlier that day [and back home] it presented a ray of sunshine to grab onto the hope he laid out for my prospective treatment. Before we left the room I had consented to give the chemotherapy a shot [no pun intended]. Dr. Logothetis wanted us back in Houston for pre-admission tests by March 1, 1989. That timetable gave us the next four days to get home, arrange for the kids to be taken care of and put all of our financial affairs in some degree of order. We had four days to make arrangements covering the next six months!

Karen had already made up her mind she was staying in Houston with me. Although I tried to convince her to remain in Michigan with the kids, she would not hear of it. I think this was the toughest decision of her life. She had devoted her maternal talents for the last 17 years to raising our children and providing a good home with lots of love. Karen never complained or second-guessed her decision, but I sensed as we went back to the hotel to pack for home, the coming separation was a heavy burden that she could not remove from her mind.

Friday, February 24, 1989 was one of the longest days of my life. In the hotel room that night we called our family and told them we were on our way home as soon as we could catch a plane. We still didn't have much solid information to give everyone other than I had okayed chemo if that's what Doctors Cox and Logothetis agreed was necessary. I attempted to pray that Friday night but it just didn't feel right. Saying prayers for others seemed natural but in my own behalf it made me feel like a hypocrite. I settled for telling Karen that I was grateful we'd finally found a couple of doctors who DIDN'T look at me like I was already dead. She agreed and we both clung to that thought as we prepared to head back home to Michigan.

Chapter 4

LAST MINUTE ARRANGEMENTS

It's always great to get back home, and this was certainly no exception. The homecoming was sweeter than usual because Karen and I realized it could be quite awhile before we might see our kids and respective families again. The possibility of our extended absence made each minute at home with the kids very special. Even though we were honest and told them that mom and dad could end up being in Texas for a few months, I don't think the kids really understood. They didn't want to believe that the cancer I was fighting was life threatening. At this point, they had not grasped that good ol' dad might not be with them in the near future if he didn't get some help soon. I tried to explain that we didn't want to be separated from home but Houston, Texas was the only place offering the kind of help I apparently needed. It bothered Karen and me MORE than anyone else that we were going to be six states away from our home and kids. We realized right from the start that five kids in this day and age was a tremendous amount of responsibility to ask or expect from anybody...even family.

Both of us were in perpetual motion from dawn to dusk. Karen's mom and dad volunteered for the first shift of watching our five children. This was quite a commitment because they lived in East Tawas, Michigan and it was 120 miles to travel south and stay at our home with the kids. It was important to us that the kids remain together under one roof. Plus, with it being in the middle of the school year it would be much simpler to ask relatives to "children sit" in our home rather than farm the kids out to different homes. We agreed it was very significant that they at least remain in familiar surroundings. With surrogate parents a necessity, we strongly felt the kids needed the security of their own home. This would help them cope with some of the other drastic changes occurring in their lives because of their dad's cancer crisis.

On Tuesday, February 28, 1989 we were once more headed back to Houston via a 727 Southwest Airlines jet. While at home, Karen and I had split the duties of making last minute arrangements. She handled the kids and house responsibilities while I handled finances and work obligations. We had accomplished as much as possible and yet, we both realized there would be areas we overlooked. Accepting this fact, both of us started to concentrate on the task ahead.

We landed late that night at Houston Hobby airport and immediately headed for the Anderson Mayfair Hotel. The tentative schedule was for pre-admission tests the next two days and then a Friday, March 3rd consultation with Dr. Logothetis. Both of us sorely needed some rest after the schedule we had maintained at home but we were unconsciously focused towards the Friday appointment. After all, we still did not know the final diagnosis of my cancerous tumor. Was it lymphoma, sarcoma or non-seminoma? Would I have to undergo radiation, chemotherapy or both? We were aware of the possibilities but not the final determination. My medical protocol was very much in our thoughts as we waited for March 3, 1989 to arrive.

Friday came with little hoopla and much anticipation. Station #17 was again extremely crowded as our turn came to see Dr. Logothetis about 4:30 p.m. that afternoon. From the many faces we watched come and go it was apparent that he had an immense patient workload. Despite this obvious workload, he gave the impression once again that our session would not conclude until all our questions had been answered to the best of his ability. Following another brief physical examination he ushered us down the hall to a small room where x-rays and C.A.T. scans were read. As he was hanging negatives from the C.A.T. scan tests he informed us, "The shared opinion is that you have a rare form of testicular cancer called non-seminoma. We are going to administer large doses of chemotherapy and try to shrink the tumor as we kill it. Although everyone does not agree, Dr. Cox and I are leaning towards this diagnosis." Karen quickly asked, "Who disagrees with the diagnosis?"

Just as quickly, Dr. Logothetis answered, "The pathology department is not convinced because this particular type of tumor indicates a mixture of cell types."

"How big is the tumor and why do I have so much d-mn pain?" I asked abruptly.

Logothetis smiled and patiently answered, "The tumor mass is approximately 15 centimeters by 8 centimeters. Your pain is probably due to the location. It is wrapped around the bottom of your spine and pinching the large veins that run alongside your spine. These veins are called the aorta and vena cava. They supply your arteries with blood for circulation. Most of your pain, Richard, is because the tumor is pushing on your lower spine and trying to cut off the blood supply to and from your legs."

As he finished this explanation he pointed to the C.A.T. scan negatives suspended from the wall. "This pear shaped, dense mass you see is the tumor. It envelops the base of your spine and is threatening your intestines, bowels and right kidney. We need to start chemotherapy immediately to stop the growth and kill the tumor."

My mind raced as I realized that this "picture" of my insides showed the tumor extremely close to infringing on my vital organs. Studying the cross-section view of the C.A.T. scan negative my main concern unconsciously escaped my mouth with the question, "Will it shrink?"

With deadpan honesty, Logothetis said, "There are no guarantees, Richard. We hope the tumor will reduce in size as the chemotherapy drugs attack the mass. The least we are shooting for is that it will stop the growth. Again, we need to start your treatment as soon as possible. I'd like to begin the first treatment this coming Monday."

I had one more question which had been bothering me since first hearing the term back at FOH in Flint, Michigan. I hesitantly asked, "What does cancer in the fourth stage mean?"

Dr. Logothetis reassuringly smiled as he answered, "This is the medical term utilized to denote how far along the cancer is developed. It also implies the rate of growth for the malignancy. But don't worry about that right now..." I interrupted him here and inquired, "How many stages are there?" He hesitated then replied, "Four, Richard."

As this bleak information registered in my mind I just shook my head indicating I understood. The message was all too clear that I was medically considered in the last phase of cancer development. Apparently, the fifth stage was funeral arrangements.

Our conference lasted a few more minutes. Karen and I asked more questions and Dr. Logothetis gave more answers. The fact was, that as much as I dreaded the idea of consenting to chemotherapy, my choices were down to none. I'd already agreed at our first meeting that I would take the chemo drugs if absolutely necessary. Well, Dr. Logothetis did not leave much doubt as to the necessity. We left station #17 on Friday, March 3rd understanding that I was fighting for my life and about the only guarantee we had was that chemotherapy was going to be a tedious nightmare. This was also when I finally admitted to myself that my cancer battle was not going to be resolved in a few short weeks. It was indeed a fight to the finish and I now understood there was no time limit on the rounds.

Chapter 5

INTRODUCTION to CHEMOTHERAPY

Before one drop of chemotherapy drugs ever coursed through my veins, I had two major stumbling blocks constantly on my mind. One: would chemotherapy physically weaken me to the point where I could lose my will to fight? Two: if I made it through the chemotherapy treatments, where was the guarantee that the drugs would indeed stop or kill the tumor growing inside me?

These negative thoughts held me like a vise as Karen and I retreated from the M.D. Anderson facility and made the short walk back to our hotel room at the Mayfair. The same overwhelming feeling of complete helplessness gripped me that had saddled my mind so often in the last 17 days. The reality that I had no control over these circumstances was as depressing as it was frustrating. Again, I was accustomed to controlling situations; not allowing situations to control me. What could I do to help myself? When and where would it all end? I did not have the answers but I was about to get some help from an unfamiliar, yet welcome source.

Neither of us felt like eating and we knew it was going to be a long weekend before I was officially admitted to M.D. Anderson Cancer Clinic on Monday. The kids and the rest of our immediate family were anxiously awaiting our call home. Before we left Michigan we had informed them that Friday was *D-Day*. "D" for diagnosis. Karen picked up the phone and dialed home to Michigan as I decided to go down to the hotel front desk and pick up our mail.

Karen made all the calls that night. Customarily, she opened most of our mail so I left it on the phone table when

I returned from the lobby. Even during those early days of displacement we received a lot of supportive mail from friends and relatives. We'd only been back in Houston for 3 days and there were already 12-13 letters waiting in our mail bin.

One of the letters we received that night was from Don Neuville, our pastor at Linden Presbyterian Church, whom you were introduced to back in *Chapter Two*. Don's letter was short but full of his usual sincere compassion and well wishes. I think that without actually experiencing the circumstances himself, Don understood better than anybody our suffering. Don was special to both of us; but it's worth repeating that his empathy put him especially close to Karen's heart. In his letter, he gave us four verses from the Bible that he thought fit our spiritual needs and would boost our morale.

Karen looked up all four verses in our hotel supplied Bible and read them to me. When finished, she marked the places and laid the Bible on the coffee table near where I was sitting. Late that evening I picked up the Bible and began to read for myself the places Karen had marked. To be honest, reading scripture quotations was foreign to me. In the last 26-27 years of my life I'd sort of come to the conclusion that only "bible thumpers" went around reading and quoting scripture. These were all New Testament readings and vaguely I recalled that during my elementary parochial school days my preference was for the Old Testament. Between characters like Adam and Eve, Moses, Samson, David and Goliath, etc., I remembered the Old Testament as a kind of collection of "Christian fairy tales." The only thing in the New Testament that interested me was Revelations. That captured my slight attention because it was purported to reveal the end of the world. If the end was coming, I figured it was my husbandly and parental obligation to know about it. I had attempted to read that two or three times and finally concluded that the author had misnamed Revelations. Because of the language and symbolism I felt something like "Divine Concealments" would have been more appropriate.

Please don't misunderstand me. I believed in God and also believed that no matter what denomination we hung our hat under we were all praying to the same God. Most important to MY beliefs was the idea that good people would go to heaven. Naturally, I assumed, that despite some small personality quirks, I was basically a good human being. Therefore, my heavenly seat MUST be reserved. I'm not certain how God considered my earthly status but it was a foregone conclusion to me — good people [even the *near good* ones] went to heaven.

I read and reread all four scripture quotes that night. I really tried to draw some strength from those ancient words. One quote captured my attention, I persisted in studying it because the verse seemed to fit my needs during these helpless days and nights. The verse was from the New Testament *John 16:33:*

These things I have spoken unto you, that in me ye might have peace. In the world ye shall have great tribulation, but be of good cheer: for I have overcome the world.

I memorized this verse that night and repeated it over and over to myself trying to comprehend its meaning. The words "ye might have peace" seemed to offer a portion of what my mind needed to contend with this cancer threat. And yet, I didn't need to "overcome" the whole world...just cancer. My instinct told me there was definitely something in those words to grab onto but I couldn't seem to grasp the full meaning. This was the first time since my battle with cancer began that I had looked for outside help. This "outside" help was truly an unfamiliar, but welcome source. I had forgotten how to communicate with God when I was around 13 years old and had neglected to try most of the time since. Remember, I evolved from a climate of complete self-reliance; the dogma that "if I can't do it, nobody can." This concept makes for great self-esteem [notice I did not say healthy self-esteem] but also carries many sleepless nights with the self-appointed badge. Cancer stole this complete self-reliance from me; how could I combat something I couldn't see and didn't understand? It left me feeling totally helpless and completely out of control. The Bible verse seemed to give me an unexplainable calm, a momentary sense of relief which my emotions couldn't deny.

When I headed for bed it was after 2:00 in the morning. Searching my mind for the full meaning of verse *John 16:33*, I snuggled up to Karen and grabbed some fitful sleep. Before drifting off, my mind kept repeating the message that today and Sunday would be very long days. Although I was not looking forward to undergoing chemotherapy, I was well aware that I had to start before I could finish. Monday! Hurry, Monday! The scripture quotes were forgotten. God had taken a back seat again...it was up to me...just me.

CHEMOTHERAPY AS TREATMENT

Browsing back through the pages I've written so far I notice the word "first" quite a few times. These "firsts" are not meant to be redundant. Just the opposite in fact, they are meant to be accurate. Many "firsts" did occur for my wife and myself as we met cancer on its terms. The pain and side effects of chemotherapy brought many more "firsts" into our every-day lives. For some unknown reason Karen and I both kept daily journals during my courses of chemotherapy. This fact was not a pre-arranged agreement. It just happened. In retrospect, I think the journals helped alleviate the monotonous hospital routine and provide some meaning in our new environment. Recording our private impressions seemed to diminish some of the frustration as we tried to accept the unending, abrupt changes.

With the assistance of both journals, I've chosen to share our candid entries and give the reader a first-hand look at the routine of chemotherapy sessions. The daily grind may have a repetitive ring to it in some places. Often, the days were similar to one another, but in fact, no two days were alike. The uniqueness lies in the perception of daily events through my eyes and Karen's, not just the actual treatment.

For any cancer patients currently undergoing chemotherapy treatment, or about to, please read the next couple of
chapters with an open mind. My intention is not to scare or
discourage anyone. Rather, my intention is to be honest
about the treatment itself and the different emotions that
coincided with it. REMEMBER, no two cancer patients are
going to react to chemotherapy the exact same way. We are
all different. Some people will be more susceptible to specific
chemo drugs than others. Some people will have more tolerance to certain chemo drugs than others. The bottom line is
that this is MY story. Therefore, any side effects or discomfort
I share with you on these pages are only an indication of MY
tolerance and susceptibility. Again, the session by session
sharing of my specific chemotherapy treatments is not intended to frighten any patients, spouses, friends or relatives.
Conversely, my aim is to remove "fear of the unknown" by
familiarizing you with chemotherapy through my personal
experience. I survived chemotherapy and SO CAN YOU.
With an open mind, the worst that can happen by reading on
is that you will have a basic understanding of the drugs and
treatment.

Let's face facts: from a medical standpoint, the treatment
has to be stronger than the disease. With cancer, the disorgan-
ized cells that make up a malignant tumor are extremely
resistant to "normal medicine." Therefore, it takes a drug that
is indeed more potent and powerful than the cancer mass
itself — meaning the toxic drugs and application we call
chemotherapy — to treat cancer. In simple terms, the medical
world has learned the hard way that when dealing with
cancer you have to fight fire with fire. Bluntly speaking, I feel
it's a matter of fighting cell poison [cancer] with drug poison
[chemotherapy].

It was almost noon on Monday, March 6, 1989 when I was
officially admitted as a non-resident [i.e.non-Texan] patient
at M.D. Anderson Cancer Clinic. My records were lost so
Karen and I were delayed about two hours in getting to our
9th floor private room. The very first thing that caught our
attention was that I stood out like a sore thumb because I had

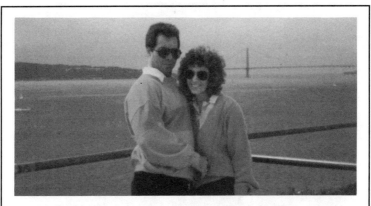

October 1988, Karen and me vacationing in San Francisco four months before the tumor in my abdomen is discovered.

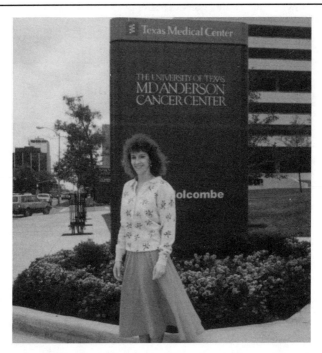

Karen waiting for me by the entrance sign on the concourse in front of M.D. Anderson.

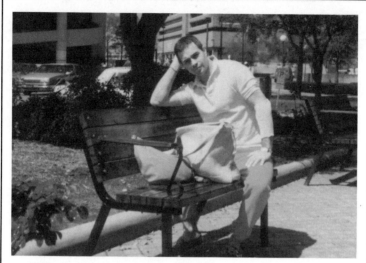

Sitting in front of the Lutheran building and enjoying the warm, Houston sun before starting chemotherapy.

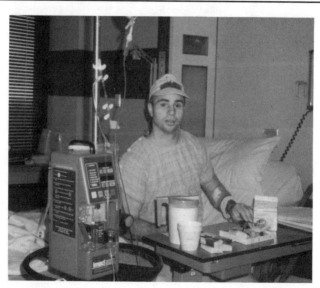

Getting ready to record more journal entries at my makeshift, bedside workstation during first chemotherapy treatment.

hair on my head. Every other patient on the 9th floor was as bald as a cue ball. No one had to tell either of us what predicated the "egghead" look. Chemotherapy left no doubt who the cancer patients were. We had also learned to detect the tell-tale signs of radiation treatment. A purplish dye marked many of these patients and that usually indicated where the tumor was located which was being bombarded with radiation. For clarity sake, you should know that my floor was all chemo patients. Every patient on the 9th floor was currently undergoing some form of chemo treatment.

Our number one priority after being admitted was to begin searching for an apartment where we could go between chemo sessions. Although Karen could live right in our private room with me while I was hospitalized, we knew that at some point I would be an out-patient. This situation demanded that we acquire a home away from home. Two households to maintain [Houston and Michigan] was not financially appealing, but it was necessary. Karen was handed this responsibility so all my concentration and energy could be channeled towards preparing for the chemo treatment which I was scheduled to begin the following day. Like many other housing problems which would pop-up later, Karen handled this one in fine fashion. With the help of her brother, Steve, [who had just spent two days driving my car from Michigan down to Houston for us] she managed to obtain a reasonably priced apartment that was less than three miles from the M.D. Anderson facility. The apartment complex provided a shuttle bus to and from the hospital once every hour from 7:00 a.m. until 5:00 p.m., five days a week. This filled our immediate needs. Steve helped move our belongings into the new apartment and that eliminated one more area of distracting pressure and concern.

Apartment hunting was now behind us, so in good conscience, it was time to worry about the chemo again. I'd had hundreds of needles poked into me in the last three weeks, the next step was to allow one more with the implanting of a permanent line into my left arm. In essence, this replaced the necessity of any temporary I.V. [intravenous] lines. This "permanent" line was called a CVC [central venous catheter] and would be with me for the duration of treatment. The CVC is designed to get drugs into the patient's bloodstream without requiring a new needle poke for an I.V. line each time. I also heard the CVC line referred to as a shunt or medport. Under any name, it was virtually indispensable. The strongest of veins cannot take the daily needle pokes and constant flow of drugs which chemotherapy demands without breaking down eventually.

In a minor bedside surgery, two capable nurses from the Infusion Therapy Team performed the procedure. My arm was locally frozen before they made a small incision for the catheter line. Next, they pushed a thin, hollow, plastic line into a large vein on the inside of my left arm [below the elbow]. Carefully guiding it the length of my arm, through my shoulder and down to my heart. This precise CVC procedure required special training for the Infusion Therapy nurses because among other things, a lung can be punctured very easily as the line is implanted.

The intravenous line can also be placed below either collarbone versus using the arm for a transport. Transport is a term used to identify the function of the plastic line which artificially replaces the patient's vein. The central venous catheter is literally a "transport" for the chemo drugs to be carried into and through the patient's veins without breaking down those veins. The drugs can be pumped or gravity flowed through this line. The CVC was definitely a relief to my worn out veins.

After settling into our hospital room, I had a lot of time to meditate and just plain think. The irony of this situation was that now I had so much time on my hands and before I had gotten sick that was just what I never had enough of...TIME. Time to a hospital patient can be very self-destructive. The wait, watch, and listen routine of a hospital allows too much opportunity for the patient to have a personal pity party.

In my opinion, self-pity, obsessive negative thoughts and ordinary laziness can all lead to long range problems for ANY hospital patient. Not just hospitalized cancer patients. These negative emotions can literally inhibit our white blood cells' immune fighting capacity by undermining the physical recuperative powers of the human body. To me, it was a matter of injecting my mind with positive thoughts and images in hopes of promoting positive body response. The very first area I attacked with positive attitude was chemotherapy. I told myself that I needed chemo, it would help me beat cancer and that I could handle whatever dosages were required. I tried to put my mind in line with the words coming from my mouth and hoped my body heard the positive interaction. Personally, I tried to recognize the symptoms of self-pity and combat them before they ever got a foothold. It wasn't easy and it ISN'T easy...but it is essential. Again, I'm wholeheartedly convinced that keeping your mind and body as busy as possible will take you a long ways in assisting your own recovery. I labeled this kind of "keeping busy" as a PAR. It's my own term, and stands for *Positive Action Routine*.

A CASE OF THE "Oh, Gods!"

As I prepared for chemo I wasn't just worried about my physical welfare. My mind wandered and worried over anything and everything. It appears to be a human characteristic to want to be in control. Control is knowledge. Control is leverage. Control is power. When we can't have that old control switch operating, our mind seems to take over and begin sending distress signals to the rest of our anatomy. Well, I can be an extremely good worrier when I really get into the worry mode. My mind can contemplate all kinds of negative notions when a situation or circumstance is out of my control.

My journal notes remind me that March 6th is the date I fretted myself into one of those penetrating "worry modes." Alone with my thoughts and having all this time on my hands, I fell into some pretty deep reasoning that Monday afternoon. One line of heavy thinking kept entering my mind. It was the concept that over the years I had heard the exclamation "Oh, God!" from so many different people under so many different circumstances, including myself. I'd heard it expressed in conversation, in the newspapers, on radio and TV, even in sports events. I'd heard it at home, at work, at play.

Sitting on the edge of my hospital bed, I pondered all the occasions I had heard human beings calling on help from God. I wondered what made us think, as human beings, that we had the right to call on God's assistance ONLY when we needed him, when the situation or dilemma we faced was out of our control. It doesn't require a genius to understand that I was in one of those out of control situations and was doing the same thing...quietly asking our benevolent God for help.

Preparing for chemotherapy was definitely pushing me towards a mild case of the *"Oh, Gods!"*

I was in a pensive mood as I debated why we ran to God when our life was out of synch and looked skyward to rectify all kinds of trouble. It occurred to me how I'd heard "Oh, God" expressed in about every imaginable context of human emotion. From anger to ecstasy to fear; and from passion to despair to elation. Over the years, I think I'd heard them all in one form or another.

For instance: What does the man say who is trapped in his wrecked car and waiting to be rescued? He's accidentally run off the road and struck a tree. The rescue team is using the jaws of life in an attempt to free him from the wreckage. He is bleeding internally and has broken bones. What does he say? He pleads, "Oh God, help me! Please help me!" How many times have we read a similar account in our local newspapers or during the course of a magazine article? We call on our unseen God and ask him to save us. For once, we probably don't even tell him how, we just want to be rescued and live. "Use your imagination God, but get me out of here and out of harm's way."

And how about the single parent mom who arrives home to find her house is enveloped in flames and her sleeping children are trapped inside? She frantically shrieks, "Oh God Oh God, help me get my children out!" It's a natural response to a critical situation. It's also an admission that in some things only our unseen God may be able to help.

What does the combat infantryman say to himself as he

lays pinned down by enemy fire with rounds ricocheting and zinging over his head? He makes a pact with God. He promises to walk a much straighter path as he implores, "Oh God, help get me out of here. Just get me away from these bullets. I'm not ready to die." How many men have thought or spoken these words? I can answer this one — *too* many good men because we've had *too* many bad wars. We look to that unseen God and ask for one of his small miracles.

What does the housewife say who just found out her husband has lost his job and fifteen years of seniority to a plant closing? They have two small children and recently purchased their long-awaited dream home. She pleads her case with an, "Oh God, what are we going to do?" The scene is probably enacted in some home, in some town or city, in some state of the U.S. every single day. We look to that unseen but ever present God and ask him to solve our crises.

Finally, what does the man, woman or child say who has just been told they have cancer? I'm quite sure that at some point they say something similar to, "Oh God, not me!" Or maybe the exclamation, "Oh God, it can't be!" Our mind says it whether our mouth does or not. Because once again our unseen God is the only source we can turn to and ask for intervention.

Common pleas for uncommon circumstances; the kind of circumstances which we are humanly helpless to change. We can combat cancer but we can't change the fact that we have contracted the disease. The word cancer has a terminal connotation to it and a feeling of total helplessness is the human emotion that goes with the diagnosis. Why else would we need God's assistance? If the situation were within our human control we certainly would not be calling on God. At least, I wouldn't. I always figured he'd be there *If and When I Needed Him*. Sounds kind of one-way now that I've admitted this short-sighted relationship.

This mild case of the *"Oh, Gods"* was a forerunner of things to come. As you read the next couple of chapters, be aware that there is a subtle transition taking place. I'm gradually moving from a state of complete self-reliance and commitment to medical treatment towards one of accommodation.

Most of the transition is a quiet change in my perception of what this cancer struggle is REALLY all about. What I begin to discover as I trudge through these initial two courses of chemotherapy is that the assurances I'm looking for are not possible. I am seeking GUARANTEES. The kind of emotional and mental guarantees that offer immunity to spreading and reoccurrence of cancer. The kind of guarantees that allow one to calmly smile through each day and peacefully sleep through each night. What I now understand is that the peace I endeavored to find is only available through faith. My faith, based on my belief, in a higher authority over life and death — faith in the unseen God of the Bible.

Chapter 6

CISCA II:
THE FIRST COURSE
of CHEMOTHERAPY

It's time to explain what a session of chemotherapy consists of in medical terms. Sessions and courses are synonymous when referring to chemotherapy treatments. A course [or session] consists of a cycle of selected chemo drugs and the amount of time it takes to intravenously feed them into the bloodstream. The cycle is repeated a minimum of 21 days apart and that minimum is utilized only if the patient's blood counts are recovered to a relative safe point. Blood count is medically defined as the number of red and white corpuscles contained in a given volume of blood. For my experimental chemo program, each course would consist of radical strength drugs administered every 21 days in large doses. Maybe this explains why I had to sign release papers before I could participate in the experimental control group.

Specifically, my first course of chemo was called Cisca II. This is a combination of three drugs which are administered intravenously, in sequence, continuously, for approximately 72 hours. Cisca II is comprised of cytoxin, adriamycin, and cisplatin. The sequence scheduled for me was cytoxin, adriamycin, cytoxin again, adriamycin again, then finish up with the "fun one" — cisplatin.

JOURNAL ENTRIES
•*DAY 1: TUESDAY, MARCH 7, 1989 — 2:20 P.M.*
This is D-Day. The chemo drugs will be humming through

my I.V. lines soon. I've had all the comparison tests and am now itching to get started so I [we] can get finished. NEWS FLASH: Before I forget, received many beautiful cards today but my mom's and sister Lisa's were special. Karen Marie and I agree that these cards from home keep us going. I'm feeling more and more, as the days go on, that I have to put my trust in God and make my contribution with a positive attitude and good body maintenance. Easier said than done.

3:30 P.M. — Chemo not here yet! Hope to record more in my journal before going to bed.

5:15 P.M. — Karen thinks it has been a depressing day. The constant changes and many adjustments are hard on us both. She says she would like to wake up tomorrow and find out that the last month has just been a terrible nightmare and have all this despair disappear. She knows God must have a plan but she wouldn't wish this on anyone. She reminds me often that we are still blessed with five beautiful children and our loving, caring families. We both realize we couldn't manage back home without the help of our parents and siblings. Still, when I see the anguish and pain etched in her face as right now, it's not easy for me to remember to count our other blessings.

7:00 P.M. — I've finally started my first course of Cisca II. I expect to get sick immediately and yet am trying not to anticipate the effects of the drugs. This is difficult because the Oncology department at M.D. Anderson provides each chemotherapy patient with a written pamphlet naming some of the possible side effects. I read it yesterday but the memory is still fresh in my mind. The pamphlet also provides a basic explanation of the drugs and their application. The information is helpful but at the same time somewhat confusing. The confusion centers around the fact that reading about possible side effects comes up short in comparison to actually experiencing side effects. By listing some of the known side effects it leaves the door wide open for human nature to take over and start to anticipate some of those side effects. Seems like a *Catch-22*. To know is to understand and yet not REALLY knowing is to anticipate. My own remedy for the dilemma is to try to keep busy.

9:45 P.M. — Almost three hours of chemo and I still feel fine. Miss the kids already. Hope they are doing fine at home. Dr. Logothetis says we need the tumor to shrink so that's what I'm concentrating on with visualization exercises. These exercises consist of mentally picturing [mental imagery is the technical term] the breakdown and dissolvement of the large tumor located in my abdomen. Takes relaxed concentration and some degree of imagination. Getting very tired. Goodnight and think shrink!

•DAY 2: WEDNESDAY, MARCH 8, 1989 — 8:30 A.M.
The first night of my first course of chemo was relatively uneventful. The severe back pain from the tumor around the base of my spine and against my vena cava remains unchanged. My lower right abdomen is still swollen and full of pressure. I still feel contaminated with the tumor inside me. Added to these constants is the new companion I've acquired...the I.V. pump and roller stand. Wherever I go, so goes the I.V. pole. Makes it very difficult to sleep or rest but it is starting to grow on me as I push or pull it everywhere. Getting into and out of the bathroom definitely takes some getting used to with my new found companion. The lab drew blood from me about 6:00 a.m. The nurses came in four times through the night and checked my vital signs [temperature, blood pressure and pulse]. They also monitor the chemo bags hanging from the I.V. pole as they take vitals. I asked a nurse about this and she said they are checking the pump rate, the I.V. site in my arm, and the I.V. lines [coming from the pump] for air pockets. Standard procedure, I guess.
11:10 A.M. — Karen is walking stiff this morning. She says the chair that folds into a bed is going to take some getting used to; it's really uncomfortable for her back. Just like her, she seldom complains. She's already noticed that we are not going to get much sleep with the nursing staff checking my vital signs as often as they do. That's good for me [in the long run anyway] and bad for her — she needs rest. Especially with all the stress she is handling. Got a lesson in medical technology yesterday which might be newsworthy. For some reason, I'd thought spreading and metastasizing meant the

same thing. They do not. Spreading infers that the tumor itself expands or stretches out while metastasizing means that the tumor jumps to other locations somewhere in the body. In other words, the primary tumor can emit another tumor in a different location of the body by using the bloodstream or lymphatic system to get there. Medically, metastasis appears to be the worst of the two. My stomach is queasy again but I'm going outside and walk. Although it is sunny the sky looks cold and windy. Just noticed that we have a room with a view. We can see the hospital parking ramp and lot. Isn't THAT special!

5:45 P.M. — My temperature is up and I just threw up. The upchucking doesn't appear to have settled my stomach down. Am going down to the Activity Room and ride the stationary bike for awhile. Want to keep moving plus Karen can work on one of those 1,000 piece jigsaw puzzles. Seems to take her mind off me and the hospital routine. The Activity Room is on our floor. It has a running machine, the bike, TV, card table and lounge chairs. Looks to me like more of the spouses use this small facility than the patients. At least it's available.

8:20 P.M. — Just finished an evening walk around the whole front of the M.D. Anderson complex. Karen went with me. We figure the sidewalk route we took is over a quarter mile but under a half mile. Went around three times. Cracks in the sidewalk are tough on the rubber wheels of my I.V. cart. The fresh air felt good but the elevator ride down, and then back up, made me dizzy and played havoc with my stomach. The hospital food that is brought to our room on plastic serving trays makes me instantly sick to my stomach. Chemotherapy has apparently heightened my sense of smell and made me very susceptible to odors. Talked to Karen about it and we're going to ask them to leave the tray outside the room tomorrow. Remember the stationary bike ride I took earlier this evening? Well, I did fine for about 30 minutes, then I caught the I.V. line on the bike pedal and nearly yanked the CVC out of my left arm. My conscience, I mean Karen, was working a jigsaw puzzle as she glanced over and said, "Let that be a lesson to you." I'm not positive but I think Oliver Hardy once said the exact same words to Stan Laurel [I'm an admitted Laurel and Hardy buff]. Seemed a lot funnier during their exchange. However, it was a lesson and I did acknowledge that I would be a little more careful during any future exercise biking. This slight incident sufficed as our excitement for the day. Until tomorrow, think shrink.

•DAY 3: THURSDAY, MARCH 9, 1989 — 8:00 P.M.

I'm starting to have bouts of nausea and get small earaches and am only about halfway through the infusion of this treatment. Have had severe stomach cramps since early this a.m. It doesn't help my nausea when every time I look at the I.V. pole the bag of adriamycin reminds me of a bottle of Gatorade. Very unsettling to a queasy stomach, thinking about that whole bag of orange, Gatorade looking drugs going into your body. I've probably drank worse stuff over the years but it just doesn't seem the same to my stomach. At this point, I've been given cytoxin twice, and this is my second 24 hour dose of adriamycin. I'm not as sick as I imagined I'd be — but I'm not feeling as good as I let on either. Have made up my mind to talk positive at all times, regardless of how I actually feel. This third day of chemo I'm getting to practice my PAR [Positive Action Routine] quite a bit. Whether I want to or not, must maintain positive actions to support positive thoughts and words. Feel strongly that it is the key to helping myself.

10:00 P.M. — The stomach cramps are still quite intense. The doctors think that the tumor is reacting violently to the chemo drugs. Hence, all the stomach pain, diarrhea and nausea. Karen says I'm a baby about the enemas I'm having to take. That's okay, she's probably right. The fact remains, no more enemas please! I might add, whoever said enemas are supposed to make you feel better is crazy. Cisplatin, the last drug for this course of chemo, is scheduled to be hung soon. This is the "fun one" which makes everyone so very sick according to our floor nurses and some of the other patients. Good! I can't wait. Just want to get this first session over with. Can't sleep, but am trying to visualize the tumor shrinking. Have haunting, black thoughts dominate my night times. Seem obsessed with thoughts of spreading and reoccurrence. Furthermore, it seems I'll have to add metastasizing to that vein of dark thoughts due to the new found separation of terms. Peace of mind is just a phrase on nights like this. I feel all alone against cancer when the lights go off. My mind is an unwilling captive to these negative perceptions. My only defense is to consciously resist the ugly notions and refuse to let cancer bully my mind into submission. God, did I ever take good health for granted. What happened? Until tomorrow, goodnight.

•DAY 4: FRIDAY, MARCH 10, 1989 — 4:30 P.M.

What a night...and what a morning! About midnight they hung cisplatin on my I.V. pole. By 3:00 a.m. I was throwing up very hard and about 15 minutes apart. Would finish vomiting, crawl back to bed, just get settled and the next round of vomiting would begin. Karen says that the marathon vomiting lasted well over six hours. At 9:15 a.m. this morning I had the last spell of throwing up. I say I went to sleep then...Karen says that I collapsed from exhaustion. Either way, my body had taken about all it could and needed rest. Karen was a saint. She held my head, got me to and from the bathroom, and babysat me all through this nasty episode with cisplatin. Neither of us was prepared for the severity of the vomiting and diarrhea. I know I wasn't. The cramps don't seem to let up BUT, I just realized, the fist-clenching back pain that has progressively gotten worse for the last 7-8 months is GONE. Hallelujah and thank God for small miracles. I had begun to wonder if I would ever again have an hour without that excruciating back pain. Am still feeling awfully weak. Will try to record more before we call it a day and go to bed. Am going to see a patient I met yesterday who's taking the same treatment as me. His name is Eddie "T". He's on the same floor but opposite wing.

8:10 P.M. — Karen taking alot of calls from home. Family and friends checking up on us. It's a point of contact with our "old life" so we both enjoy the phone conversations. Each hospital room has a telephone and its own private number for incoming and outgoing calls. Tonight, Karen's handling the phone duties for both of us. My memory is fuzzy regarding last night's events. What I do recall of the cisplatin experience is not pleasant. Am still very weak from the whole ordeal. Cramps, diarrhea and fatigue continue to grip me. About 7:00 p.m. I forced myself to go outside and walk around the complex twice. My I.V. pole felt as if it weighed a half ton. The walk was tiring but the air put some color back into my face. Not much spring in my walk yet. By the way, had a nice visit with Eddie "T". Hails from Missouri now but he was originally born and raised in Texas. He is on his second course of chemo and is being treated for testicular non-seminoma. Eddie wasn't sure what type of non-seminoma cancer he had been diagnosed with. To tell the truth I don't think he wanted to know what category his tumor fell into. As we chatted, I got the distinct feeling that the more I desired to know about cancer the less he wanted to know. Guess everyone copes in different ways. Eddie admits to being apprehensive. I think scared would be more accurate and that description fits all of us that are combatting cancer. Surprisingly, he has not lost any hair to the chemo treatments yet. Every other patient on this floor, except me, is bald. From what I hear, pretty soon I WON'T be able to say those words.

10:35 P.M. — It appears that I've traded the back pain for gut-wrenching cramps. That's alright. One problem at a time. I'm just thankful the back pain is gone. This thing [tumor] inside me feels alive. It gurgles, hisses and rumbles like an active volcano. The stomach cramps are all across my lower abdomen and seem to get worse with each passing hour. Karen and I are both extremely tired. Will call the kids tomorrow and touch base with them when I feel better.

•DAY 5: SATURDAY, MARCH 11, 1989 — 8:05 A.M.
Didn't sleep well. Cramping pain in my stomach woke me periodically throughout the night. Couldn't keep my mind from dwelling on how helpless I feel in combatting this filthy cancer lodged in my abdomen. This is SO-O-O different than anything I've ever come up against. Always felt that any obstacle could be overcome if you applied concentration, motivation and effort to the situation. Not true when fighting

cancer. All of MY efforts bring no guarantees. The uncertainty can be terrifying and even downright disabling.

3:30 P.M. — Haven't eaten in over three days and still feel drained and dehydrated. I have no appetite and am continuing to fight nausea and diarrhea. Trying to throw up as your stomach cramps and your bowels move is not a natural condition for the human body. God designed us better than that...I think He wanted us to do one or the other, NOT both at the same time. Dr. Logothetis and his fellowship intern, Dr. Ziegler, were in early this morning. They discussed the possibility of emergency surgery if the stomach inflammation I am enduring does not let up. They're afraid of a bowel obstruction. At this point, if they are afraid then so am I. Don't know what to hope or pray for because as much as I want the tumor removed I understand that it needs to be dead tissue before the doctors can be relatively sure that surgery will get it all. Am going down for x-rays in awhile to see if there is indeed a bowel obstruction.

5:05 P.M. — Just returned from x-ray. Told Karen that it's the same scene each time I go for any testing. A group of patients wait their respective turn for the test and while we wait it seems like they all want to tell you THEIR cancer story. This pattern has repeated itself for the many tests I've had to undergo. I'm sure that sharing their particular cancer story helps these patients cope but it bothers me immensely. One story after another: from metastasizing to spreading to reoccurrence. Two middle aged men, both from Texas, came in for a routine check-up and malignant tumors were re-discovered. Both men were supposedly cured. One gentleman from Abilene, Texas had been cancer free for almost seven years and now a tumor has been found in his left lung. The other gentleman was here for his two year checkup. This man was very subdued and did not elaborate on where his specific cancer had re-occurred. I keep asking myself, why? Why do they have to fight for their lives again? It seems to help them when they tell someone, so I listen. The doctors will tell us my x-ray results in the morning. God above, please help me get some sleep tonight. I've forgotten how to really pray. Hope God still listens.

•DAY 6: SUNDAY, MARCH 12, 1989 — 10:20 A.M.
Karen looks better today, the color has returned to her complexion. She says she slept pretty good. That's great because her mind and body sorely needed the rest. My night was restless. Thanks to the terrible cramps I spent much of it gazing at the darkened ceiling of our room and worrying. I know it won't help but the negative thoughts seem to obsess my mind some nights. Letting go and admitting I can't control this situation is so very difficult for me. The lack of control brings with it real, unimagined panic. Dr. Logothetis was in around 9:00 a.m. and said the x-rays showed no apparent bowel obstruction. That was good news but the horrible cramps remain. He also said we might be able to go "home" to our apartment by Tuesday.

1:15 P.M. —Went for a long walk. When I returned Karen had all the kids, except Melissa, on the phone. We've only been gone a week and it seems like a month. All the kids sounded good. After we hung up Karen got very quiet. That's her way of coping. Some tears quietly slipped down her cheeks as she turned her head from me and stared out our 9th floor window into the adjacent parking ramp. It's awfully hard on her being away from the kids. Her daily life has centered on being a good mom for the last seventeen years and I think she feels guilty about being gone. She's a trooper. Just the same, I don't enjoy seeing her torment herself. Stacey and Randy seem to be the hardest on her emotionally because they are the youngest and she knows they need her reassuring physical presense the most during these early, formative years. I try to cheer her spirits but I can't fill that void created by our separation from the kids.

7:15 P.M. — Many calls from Michigan today. My brother Craig called first. He is having some rough days from the radiation treatments U of M Ann Arbor Hospital is administering for his cancer. No matter how difficult some of my days are, I never forget that Craig has cancer also. It's a personal battle for both of us. My old business and workplace is far down on my priority list these days but I relish being told ANYTHING from home. Even like hearing how our old, but not forgotten, employees are faring. Craig is always candid and usually spices up the events with his own dry humor. In abbreviated form his joke for the day went like this: "Didja hear about the guy who accused God of letting him die?" Naturally, I replied 'No.' "Well, he had a terminal disease and believed that God was going to heal him. His first day in the hospital a radiologist came in and told him they would like to begin radiation treatments tomorrow. The man said, 'Thanks anyway, but my God will take care of me.' The next day the head oncologist came to his room and stated they should begin chemotherapy immediately. The man replied, 'No thanks, my God will take care of me.' On the third day the chief surgeon enters his room and tells him they have surgery scheduled that afternoon. The man says, 'Thanks doc, but I don't need it. My God is going to heal me.' On the fourth day the man died and went to heaven. When he got there he informed St. Peter that he had a bone to pick with God. St. Peter said, 'No problem, at 2:00 p.m. each day God grants interviews.' This guys turn comes and he kneels down before God and says, 'Lord, with all due respect, You lied to me. You said to trust You...I did. You said believe in your words...I did. You said put my faith in you...I did. Lord, why did You ignore my prayers and let me die?' God smiled down at him and said, '*My son, I DIDN'T lie to you or ignore your prayers. WHO do you think sent the radiologist, oncologist and surgeon to see you?!*" At the punch line I laughed my head off. Told Craig that I think I got the message. Shortly after Craig hung up, Karen's parents called. Really enjoyed talking to them and loved the way their voices lifted Karen's spirits. Helen and Dean have been a great help through this ordeal. Time to go visiting. I know a couple of patients on the floor now so if the door to their room is open I usually stop in to chat. Therapy for all involved. Maybe I'll retell my brother's joke. Then again, maybe I won't since I don't know everyone's capacity for humor.

•DAY 7: MONDAY, MARCH 13, 1989 — 9:30 A.M.
It's Stacey's birthday today. She is eleven years old [our second youngest]. Stacey is having a rough time dealing with our absence so Karen and I are both trusting that her birthday

celebration chases some of the blues away. We'll call her later, sometime after school is out. Dr. Logothetis was in at 8:00 a.m. He feels that the cramps and diarrhea remain severe because the tumor is trying to resist the chemo drugs. My whole abdomen area is inflamed. Logo [as Dr. Logothetis shall hence forth be called — no disrespect intended] says the x-rays indicate that the tumor has actually enlarged a little. He explains that the enlarging is from the tumor reacting violently to the chemo. This info did NOT make my day. Here I am visualizing day and night that the tumor is shrinking and the first report we receive is that it is enlarging. The fact that it is bigger disturbs me greatly but the explanation makes sense. What it amounts to is another unexpected wrinkle to deal with and add to the often overwhelming feeling of complete helplessness. The final word from Logo was that the consulting doctors were still considering emergency surgery. I wish the cramps would ease up, even if just for awhile. Sometimes, the pain literally brings tears to my eyes.

4:40 P.M. — They are starting to feed me intravenously. The nurses came in with some white "food" in a bottle. Looks like baby formula to me. Karen says that's basically what it is. Haven't eaten in over five days so Logo is trying to supplement me with 2500 liquid calories a day. The feeding is medically referred to as hyperalimentation. My body needs the nourishment but it sure isn't the same as eating steak and potatoes. Seem to feel my worst each day in the late afternoon and early evening. Temperature usually goes up; cramps and nausea become worse. Like many other quirks it is unexplainable.

10:20 P.M. — My dad called tonight. He worries about us out here and needs to hear my voice sometimes just to nullify his own nagging doubts. We had a nice talk. I'm trying to relax and put the threat of emergency surgery completely out of my mind. Logo explained this morning that they prefer to complete chemotherapy before surgery because the tumor is well-defined and all the cell tissue is dead if chemotherapy is successful. This makes the surgery itself less risky. Anyway, am really concentrating on being positive and getting through ALL the chemo before surgery. It's difficult. The pain doesn't seem to let up and that plays on your mind after awhile. Oh well, very tired and it's time to do the positive imaging exercises that I put myself through each night. I'm still thinking SHRINK.

•DAY 8: TUESDAY, MARCH 14, 1989 — 6:00 P.M.

Another long, long day in the hospital. We try to keep busy but there are only so many things you can do when you are tied to an I.V. pole. Poor Karen. She needs to make a couple friends and get away from this depressing hospital routine once in awhile. We're meeting new people but most of them are in the same boat we are...the spouse has cancer and they also are stuck in the hospital. Karen does try to visit our apartment each day and get the mail if nothing else. When she returns from the apartment we have our own private mail call. It's always an uplifting experience to hear from our family, friends and even acquaintances from back home. We are missed and loved and the letters sustain our morale. Logo says I won't be getting out of here for a few days, still running relatively high temp in the late afternoons [around 101 degrees]. Has been raining outside all day until the sun just peeked through the clouds. I'm going for a walk, the fresh air helps give me new perspective.

•DAY 9: WEDNESDAY, MARCH 15, 1989 — 7:40 A.M.

Awoke at 5:30 a.m. as they were drawing blood. Don't sleep much as it is and could not get back to sleep after the "butcher" got ahold of my arm. This is my nickname for one of the blood team nurses. Sure she doesn't mean to but she hurts my arm when drawing blood. Hope she takes a couple days off and gives my veins a rest. Here comes my breakfast. The nurse is hanging it from my I.V. pole. They are giving me almost 3000 intravenous calories per day now. Nice balanced diet of proteins, fats and carbohydrates. I'm attempting to start eating again but can only get a few bites down without upchucking. So, until I eat on my own they will continue the I.V. feedings. Believe it or not the intravenous food actually leaves me with a satisfied, "full" feeling. Karen enjoys breakfast and would like some company. With this in mind, am certain my appetite will return soon.

2:30 P.M. — Houston, Texas is very hot and humid most of the time. Today is no exception. The weather is hazy and overcast and yet remains muggy. It's about time for the kids to get out of school back home. I think about them all through the day. Time to walk.

6:55 P.M. — My temperature got to 101.4 degrees this afternoon. Also experiencing chills and earaches. Logo ordered stool, urine and blood cultures to be taken. In addition, he started me on an antibiotic. We are kind of expecting Dr. James Cox to drop in to see us tonight. When he stops by we bombard him with questions and he usually puts our minds at ease. His visits are especially good for Karen. She is listening to Dr. Bernie Siegel* tapes at the moment. He is the author of *Love, Medicine and Miracles*, a New York Times bestseller written about cancer. Dr. Siegel is a practicing surgeon from upstate New York. He handles mostly cancer patients. Many of his personal experiences as a cancer surgeon are what motivated him to write his book. The book [and tapes] is aimed at helping the cancer patient cope and the attending physician to compassionately understand the patients point of view. His novel was well written and indicates that the patients have much to do with their own recovery [or non-recovery]. Karen's mom just called. Helen's phone calls always seem to have a soothing effect. Karen comes away with her spirits bouyed. They have a close mother and daughter relationship; and yet they are friends, on an equal basis. I thank God EACH night that neither Karen, nor any of our children, are going through this cancer struggle. If it had to strike someone in our family I'm glad it was me. And that "glad" is a relative one! This is one prayer where I don't have any communication problem with our God. On the 6th floor there are many young adolescents fighting different varieties of cancer. Leukemia, from what I have witnessed, is the form of cancer that strikes this age group most frequently. Watching these young kids suffer through chemotherapy and amputated limbs literally eats my insides apart. If nothing else, my visits to the 6th floor remind me of how fortunate I really am each time I wander down there and realize this could be one of our children. Don't think I could handle that. Pray to God every night that THEY never have to.

8:40 P.M. — Forced a small meal down this evening. Had been eight days without really eating and five days of I.V. feeding. After all the diarrhea in the last week and a half, now I'm constipated. Makes the cramps worse.

•DAY 10: THURSDAY, MARCH 16, 1989 — 7:35 P.M.

Today was a much better day than yesterday. Same symptoms but the cramps and earaches have let up a little. Trying to think, act and talk positive at all times. It requires a super human effort to keep your emotions on an even keel. Karen and I are with each other virtually 24 hours a day. As much as we love each other, we sometimes need private time and our own space. These close quarter circumstances test our unconditional love. Walked twice today. The sidewalk, which forms a rectangle in front of the Anderson complex, makes for a convenient walking route. The walks tire me out, yet, they revive my senses. Karen accompanies me on many of the walks and we have some very upbeat chats. Good for both of us. We miss the kids and wonder out loud quite often what they are doing right then. Am trying to get letters written to all of the kids and some "thank you's" to the numerous friends that have sent us cards. The mail is one thing we look forward to EVERYDAY. A gal from our hometown just called Karen. Her name is Paula. All of us grew up in the same neighborhood back home, as well as going to the same high school [Fenton]. Paula is married to a doctor who works right here at the M.D. Anderson facility and lives in a suburb of Houston. She and K.M. are planning on getting together this Saturday for a shopping trip. I think it will be great for Karen to get away from the hospital with some friendly company. Will call it a day on that happy note.

•DAY 11: FRIDAY, MARCH 17, 1989 — 5:00 P.M.

St. Patrick's Day! It's even celebrated in Texas. Many of the nurses are wearing green. Back home I know a couple of Irish friends [at least they think they are] who will probably be heavy into celebrating this evening. My temperature is up again. Almost 102 degrees. Logo can't explain what causes this rise in body temperature so it's a predicament I just accept. Probably a side effect from the chemo. Karen is missing the kids terribly today. Her makeup is running beneath her eyes so I know she's been crying. Some days are better than others for these abbreviated episodes where my comforting embrace is not enough. In Karen's own words, the separation becomes almost unbearable at times. She prays many times each day for the strength to accept this separation from our children.

9:25 P.M. — Stopped in to see a patient in the room next to mine. His name is Patrick "B". He related his whole cancer story to me. From the sounds of it, he has been through a tremendous amount of pain and disappointment already. What bothered me as he was sharing his story is that he has the exact same kind of cancer that I have been tentatively diagnosed with — testicular non-seminoma. He is taking chemotherapy for the second time. NOT his second course mind you, but his second time around for the whole chemo treatment. We talked quite awhile. He has alot of confidence in his doctors, yet he appears scared and overly apprehensive. I don't think he realizes that we ALL are afraid of this thing they call cancer. Will make a point of it to visit with him again. My brother Craig just called. He did not sound good at all. His throat passage is constricted from the radiation he's taking, therefore it's tough for him to talk. Time to meditate and see if I can touch base with that God I've forgotten how to talk with. Goodnight.

•DAY 12: SATURDAY, MARCH 18, 1989 — 8:00 A.M.
Started the day off with "the butcher" drawing blood from me at 5:45 a.m. Did not sleep well last night. All kinds of negative, black thoughts prevented me from relaxing and acquiring some sound sleep. It's funny, am not overly concerned about the huge tumor in my abdomen. May be naive thinking but I feel sure that the tumor WILL shrink, be surgically removed and not be a threat to invade other parts of my body. My major worries are reoccurrence, metastasizing and the idea

that Karen, or the kids, could contract this dreaded disease. In addition, never far from my subconscious thought are the terminal predictions of...*less than 90 days*...and...*less than 10% survival rate.* These are the same thoughts which literally haunt me almost every night. The cramping pain in my abdomen wakes me at all hours of the night. Once awake, I scramble for the bathroom and then return to bed only to grapple with the overpowering dark thoughts some more. Being perfectly honest with myself, I guess I'm looking for guarantees that after going through all this treatment, my family and myself will be immune to any further threat of cancer. We all know there are no such guarantees.

6:00 P.M. — Karen went shopping this afternoon with Paula, our "Fenton connection." She said it was a short shopping trip but she really enjoyed Paula's company and getting away from the hospital. I should mention at this time that I have the dubious honor of being married to the acknowledged "shopping queen" of all of lower Michigan. Karen unequivocally LOVES [or is it lives?] to shop.

8:10 P.M. — Our phone has rang non-stop for a solid hour and a half. My temp is over 102 degrees and I don't feel the greatest. Cramps, fever and headaches have been increasing since late afternoon. With the pain beginning to distract me, Karen is taking the brunt of our calls. I am vicariously sharing the conversations with family and friends. Felt great to hear from George, Carl and Ben. Three longtime friends whose sincere empathy comes ringing through each time they call. Sometimes I think my closest friends were struck harder by my cancer diagnosis than I was. I guess that's what real friendship amounts to — pure compassion. Plus, I understand that they realize by a subtle twist of fate this could be one of them lying here undergoing chemotherapy and fighting for their life. Empathy in its highest form. Signing off until tomorrow.

•DAY 13: SUNDAY, MARCH 19, 1989 — 8:00 A.M.
At 6:20 a.m. I was up and roaming the halls this morning. Rode the stationary bike for 26 minutes then came back to our room to see how Karen was doing. She says this is one of those

days that she feels like she is held together by a thread. She misses her hugs from the kids. Especially our littlest one, Randy, who loves to give his mom hugs. Encouraged her to call home and talk with the kids. For a change, we caught all of them at home and that in itself was uplifting. I think Karen feels better now. Once again, I sincerely suggested she return home to be with the kids. She won't even discuss it but remains torn between the conflicting responsibilities of wife and mother. Sometimes, the guilt I experience over this apparent dilemma is crushing.

9:05 P.M. — Karen went to the apartment this afternoon and picked up yesterday's mail. All the beautiful cards and letters are a great comfort. We would be lost without our mail from home and the telephone. Been a long day. Am going to visit a couple of the other patients and then call it a night. Karen is beat also.

•DAY 14: MONDAY, MARCH 20, 1989 — 7:30 P.M.
Talked to a few of the old-timers on the floor. These are the patients that have been in treatment the longest. They tell some real heartbreaking stories about themselves and other patients they've seen on the floor. Cecil "C" and John "T" are two of these veterans. The older you are in age the more the chemotherapy appears to tear your body resistance down. The effects are harder, last longer and strike the body quicker. I give these older fellas a tremendous amount of credit. Patrick "B", in the room next to mine, is having a rough time. Seems to be retaining body fluids as he appears bloated and depressed. He's very young [about 25 years old] and very scared. I try to cheer him up but the tumors in his back give him so much pain it keeps him from being able to concentrate on positive thoughts. He told me he's bedridden now.

9:15 P.M. — I weighed 175 pounds today. Have lost 14 pounds since this saga began. Not bad when I compare myself to other patients. Terry [mentioned earlier and truly one of my best friends] plans on coming down here to see us around March 23rd. Even though I discourage most visitors it would be fantastic to see him. Last year at this time, Terry and I were in Biloxi, Mississippi on a golf outing with 22 other guys. We played golf all day and cards most of the night. It was a three day getaway. What a difference a year makes! Ate one and a half pieces of pizza tonight. Frankly, the Texas version of pizza cannot hold a candle to our own Michigan pizza [in my humble opinion, that is]. But on the other hand, our chili can't touch the Texas four-alarm homemade chili. Trying to get my appetite back; with chemo affecting my senses of smell and taste so radically the spicy memory of pizza sounded good.

10:50 P.M. — John, a friend from Fenton, just called. He lives in a suburb of Dallas, Texas now. His job with Union Carbide brought him out here about three years ago. John, his wife Mona and two young sons seem to love their new life as transplanted Texans. Don't know how he ran down our phone number at M.D. Anderson but it was great talking about some of our antics back in high school and reliving those carefree days. Along with the usual discomforts, my hemoglobin reading came back below 9 and my stomach is bloated. Makes me feel weak and tired. Must eat to regain some strength and energy. It's an effort. Karen says I've been touchy most of the day. She insists I take the sleeping pill they offer because she feels strongly that I need a good night of real rest. Don't have much faith in pills but will try it her way.

•DAY 15: TUESDAY, MARCH 21, 1989 — 8:55 A.M.

First day of Spring! Raining and temperature is about 70 degrees here in Houston. Cramps and bouts of sweating woke me intermittently through the night. Have been awake since 5:00 a.m. trying to mentally picture the "meltdown" of this tumor inside me. I spend a considerable amount of time practicing and perfecting the visualization techniques I've created. Trying for *PAR excellence*. Makes me feel that I'm helping myself and accomplishing something. For this morning's mental meltdown I visualized a giant sunlamp flooding the tumor area with ultra violet rays. This shrivels and kills the tumor. Also, this effort helps support MY belief that MY cure is not left JUST to the doctors. Karen slept decent for a change and now we are going for a walk in the hospital.

My hair is beginning to fall out. The fallen hair is laying all over my pillow when I get up each morning. Oh well, I've convinced myself it's no big deal and reconciled myself to the fact that it will grow back eventually. Maybe bald *is* beautiful!

9:30 P.M. — Been an eventful day. Logo and his staff were in before lunchtime with some excellent news. The blood markers that they utilize to keep track of tumor size and growth have reduced considerably. Before chemotherapy my AFP count [the tumor marker I just referred to] was 381.6; this blood marker was down to 195.1 as of this morning. That means the chemo appears to be killing the tumor. Karen and I were elated. At least I am not going through all this humbling pain and suffering with no evident results. The timing was beautiful. Last night I prayed over and over to beat this cancer completely. I asked God to forgive my past negligence and to intervene in my behalf. I flat out told Him that I had too much to live for and was not ready to give up and die. Felt good to share my innermost worries with Him. People keep stopping me and asking, "Are you in remission?" Truthfully, that's the question that prompted opening the prayer pipeline last night. To me, remission is only a partial victory. Have made up my mind and set my will to achieve complete victory over this tumor and the nightmares of reoccurrence. Cancer is a massive bully. If you allow it to, it will dominate your every conscious thought. I've realized in the last few days that my life and personality could use some positive change. These changes will aid in accepting the helplessness that cancer brings with it. I'm working at believing that God meant and designed us to be healthy. My habits and lifestyle have contributed immensely to tearing down the masterful design of this human body. At 39 years old I look back on my daily life and see many warnings I disregarded. The subjection to chemotherapy and the threat of terminal cancer have made me realize what human existence is all about. Life is very fragile and comes with no guarantees of longevity. This comprehension lends credence to the fact that I took life's simple blessings for granted. That's what I'm learning — appreciation is NOW. Appreciation is enjoying each hour and each day, one at a time. Ironically, in life there is nothing more certain than death. *When* is the only uncertainty. Time to grab some shuteye.

•*DAY 16: WEDNESDAY, MARCH 22, 1989 — 8:05 P.M.*
GREAT NEWS: Terry slipped into town late this afternoon. This was a day earlier than scheduled. Karen tried to keep it a surprise but I had finagled a 4-hour pass out of Dr. Logothetis so it goofed up her plans. I couldn't figure out for the life of me why Karen was upset that we could finally leave the hospital for a few hours. Noticed she kept looking at her watch and that's what really tipped me off that something was in the air. She and Terry had originally planned on sneaking him up to our hospital room and entirely surprising me. When Karen finally broke down and told me Terry was flying in this afternoon we decided that we'd use our 4-hour pass to drive to Houston Hobby airport and *I would surprise him.* It worked. He was shocked to see me and I was ecstatic to see him. Just by being here Terry had brought with him a piece of home and our "old life". We gave him a mini-tour of Houston as we headed back to the hospital.

8:45 P.M. — NOT-SO-GREAT NEWS: Underwent another test this morning. The test was a C.A.T. scan of my lower abdomen. There were six patients ahead of me waiting for their scans when I arrived at the testing area. Couldn't help but listen as a 32 year old woman told the man next to her that she had two small children at home and the doctors had told her she had less than a year to live. She was from Oklahoma and had been battling uterine cancer for almost two years. It was sad because she appeared to have given up hope. The man told her he had some kind of stomach cancer called adenocarcinoma. I don't think that he felt much like talking but he was making an attempt to cheer her up by sharing his not-so-good prognosis. These situations always touch me deeply. They also depress me immediately. Makes me wonder where the patients are who have beat cancer. Obviously not here. From the very first test I took at M.D. Anderson this scene has seemed to repeat itself. I can only assume that I was meant to witness these discussions — for whatever reason.

9:40 P.M. — Terry went to our apartment to get some rest. He had worked a half day and then grabbed his flight to Houston. Looked pretty frazzled when he left. Karen has been down by the 9th floor elevators listening to some senior citizen musicians. The makeshift band volunteers their time and plays on a couple of occasions a year at the hospital. Eavesdropped on them as I rode the stationary bike in the Activity Room. They were really good! Played hoedown tunes with a mean fiddle and banjo. The "youngest" band member was 63 years old. Their specialty was yodeling and foot stomping, hillbilly music. Karen loved the entertainment and it was a nice break from the normal hospital atmosphere of reserved quiet. Going to read for awhile and try to unwind before attempting to sleep.

• *DAY 17: THURSDAY, MARCH 23, 1989 — 7:15 A.M.*
Tried to call my sister, Deb and brother, Ron late last night. They're both single and on the run quite a bit. Received inquisitive letters from each of them recently so wanted to phone and set their minds at ease. Could tell from their questions that they are worried about me. It is truly amazing how many negative rumors have been flying around back in Michigan. Neither Karen nor I start them, and we certainly don't add fuel to the ones already circulating, but we do spend a considerable amount of energy denying some of these rumors. At any rate, we are doing as well as possible [under the circumstances] and I wanted my brother and sister to know this fact.
9:30 A.M. — Terry got up to my room at 8:00 a.m. Said he slept decent. Karen wants him to help move our belongings to a new apartment before he flies back to Michigan. We qualified for one of the church sponsored apartments and this will help us financially. Although the apartment is much smaller in size, so is our monthly payment. Karen is relieved and happy because our rent will be about one half of what it was for our other apartment. Logo was just in for his morning rounds. We introduced him to Terry and then got down to business. Logo explained that the C.A.T. scan showed the tumor is still enlarged from the reaction to chemo drugs but appears deadened on the outside. He thinks most of my pain comes

from the tumor looping its tentacles around my bladder, bowels and intestines as it resists the chemo. Overall, this was good news as we take one day at a time for pluses or minuses. Terry enjoyed hearing for himself the update by Logo. Made him feel more comfortable about my actual condition. He worries about me like a brother. Wangled a six hour pass out of Logo. Hope I can make it that long on the outside. One of the things I want to do is get my hair cut very short so K.M. can start getting used to looking at me bald. Will lose the rest of it soon to the chemo treatment — so — at least I'll fit in with the other bald-headed patients on my floor. The nurse just unhooked me from the I.V. pole and heparin locked my line. Definition time. Heparin is a solution which prevents the I.V. line from clotting with blood. That's enough medical jargon for awhile....We're OUT OF HERE for six hours!

11:10 P.M. — Got very tired today. Cramps were quite bad by the time Karen, Terry and I headed back to the hospital. At least I got my haircut while we were out. Kept having to tell the barber to cut it shorter. Karen says it takes her back 20 years; that I look like I'm in Marine Corps boot camp again. It was good to get away from the hospital. Terry spent two hours donating platelets this afternoon. God bless him. Platelets are for clotting the dried blood. He was under the mistaken impression that he could earmark the platelets for me in case I required a transfusion down the road. He discovered AFTER they had the needle in his arm that platelets will only keep about seven days. He took the news in stride and his donation certainly won't go to waste. The process of donating involves separating the platelets from the donor's blood and then infusing the blood plasma back into the donor's blood. Many patients require platelet transfusions because chemotherapy [and leukemia] hinders the bone marrow from manufacturing its own platelets. M.D. Anderson loves to have donors like Terry. The big needle didn't even bother him...so he said anyway. Think shrink...and I don't mean psychiatrist.

• *DAY 18: FRIDAY, MARCH 24, 1989 — 9:10 A.M.*
This morning I met another patient with the same diagnosis as mine. His name is Kevin "M" and he's from Texas. We

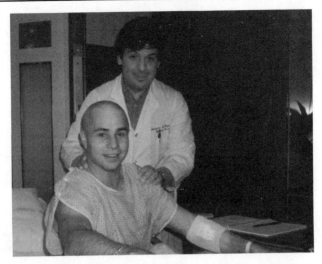

Dr. Christopher J. Logothetis, my doctor and Chief Oncologist at M.D. Anderson, making his morning rounds.

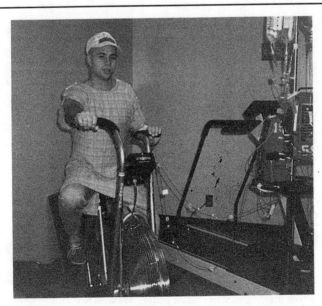

Riding the exercise bike on the 9th floor in the activity room.

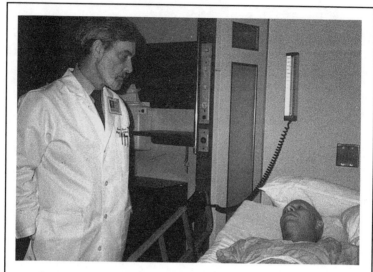

Dr. James Cox, Vice-President of Patient Affairs at M.D. Anderson, paying a social visit during chemo treatment.

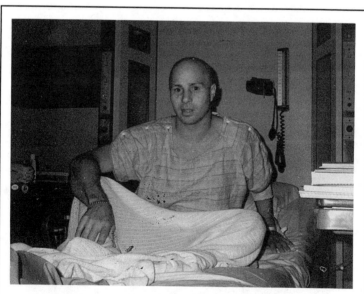

Karen making sure she had a picture of me in my bald state for her scrapbook.

traded stats and compared notes. Kevin has read a lot about non-seminoma cancer and is well informed. He has already had surgery to remove the primary tumor site. The secondary tumor is less than 3 centimeters and located near his left lung. His cancer was considered 2nd stage when diagnosed. Finally, Kevin's AFP count was at 40 when he came in for chemotherapy. He's getting ready for his second course of chemo and his sessions are 28 days apart. My talk with Kevin "M" makes me realize how advanced my cancer actually is in comparison. And that worries me considerably.

3:00 P.M. — Terry goes home on Sunday. We are watching the University of Michigan play basketball in the NCAA tournament on TV. Terry is living and dying with each basket made. He must have a bet on the game [ha ha]. Some things never change. Took him for a long walk outside and got a little sunburned while we were out there chatting. I was warned that sunburn and chemo do not mix. Will have to be careful, don't want ANY complications. Logo was in for his daily rounds. He said it is very unlikely that the tumor will shrink now. Logo still maintains that my constant cramps are caused by the tumor throwing loops around my bladder, bowels and intestines. All I know is that the pain is always there and remains extreme. Chills are beginning to get bad, that usually indicates my temperature is going up. Fits the pattern for late afternoon.

9:55 P.M. — The kids are on our minds tonight, as every night. They are kind of scattered all over for the next few days as they begin Easter vacation. Stacey and Randy are up north at their Grandma and Grandpa Ouellette's. Ricky is home packing for his eighth grade class trip to Washington, D.C. Melissa and Cheryl are headed for Florida to spend 10 days with their Grandma and Grandpa Rockman. We worry about all of them. Terry is ready to call it a day and head for our apartment. He's been great. Very tuned in to my physical condition and our situation. Doesn't expect anything and puts no pressure on us to entertain or occupy him. We're gonna miss his smiling face. Truly we are.

•DAY 19: SATURDAY, MARCH 25, 1989 — 7:40 A.M.
Good morning, H-O-U-S-T-O-N! The remark doesn't have a

lot of originality but it is a different start to an ordinary morning. My weight is holding at 175 pounds. Have been eating better and more consistent. Just looked at a computer readout on all my blood work counts. Some of them are still low; my hemoglobin for one. Logo says we will try to start 2nd course of chemo on time but the deciding factor will be my counts. At the risk of sounding like a whiner I'm still having much abdominal grief. I try not to complain but the pain is an ever present dark cloud to smile through and overcome. Could be worse, so I count my tempered blessings.

9:25 P.M. — My white blood cell count is down and my hemoglobin remains below normal. It'ş been another long, tedious day. Karen, Terry and I took two walks during the day, both of them outside. Later, I escorted Terry around our floor and introduced him to a few of the patients I've met. We didn't spend too much time in anyone's room because it made Terry feel awkward. These visits allowed him to get a glimpse of how other patients were dealing with their cancer struggle. Right now all of us are feeling the effects of a lengthy day and want to get a good night's rest. Terry flies home tomorrow and has to rise early for the flight so he's en route to the apartment intent on getting some sleep. We took the smaller church apartment and Terry promised to help move our belongings before he leaves for his airplane trip home. Karen signed papers this afternoon with the church people sponsoring this worthwhile program which assists cancer patients in finding temporary accommodations. Time to meditate. Time to relax. Time to think of how and what the kids are doing. I miss them, even their squabbling. Tomorrow is another day. Goodnight.

•DAY 20: SUNDAY, MARCH 26, 1989 — 7:35 A.M.
HAPPY EASTER! Karen Marie had a card and Easter candy waiting for me when I got out of the shower. She loves holidays. In fact, it's probably a good thing she is not president of the United States. We'd have at least one holiday a week. Since I forgot it was Easter I had to improvise and make her a card. We got choked up over each other's card message and then hugged for a long, tender moment. As we held each

other close, time and the threat of cancer seemed to momentarily stand still. While I would have liked considerably more than a hug, the hospital setting doesn't allow for any hanky-panky. Took a rain check. Karen looks absolutely gorgeous today! She's wearing a long, flowing red skirt with a new silk blouse she purchased down here. Not to mention the matching beads and earrings. Now I know how some anonymous personality coined the phrase "all dressed up and nowhere to go."

10:30 A.M. — Terry just grabbed a taxi to catch his flight from Houston to Detroit. As I said earlier, we'll both miss him. Before he left, he moved the majority of our things to the new apartment. It's definitely small compared to the other apartment. Like most everything else I'm sure we'll get used to the change. Karen phoned our two little ones at her mom and dad's home. She wanted to hear if they'd found their Easter baskets. The Easter Bunny [Uncle Dean this year] must have hid them extremely well because Stacey and Randy hunted for quite some time before discovering their baskets. Karen was upset when she finished talking and hung up the phone. Softly, with subdued control she cried for awhile. The tears seem to work as a cleansing release during these episodes of minor depression. I hate seeing Karen cry but I'm glad that she is relieving some of her pent up emotions concerning the kids. Not much I can personally do to comfort her during these times. I'm the reason she is separated from our children and I understand the complex emotions involved. Basically, seems to be a hate/love situation. She loves me or she wouldn't be here. And yet she hates me because I'm the reason she is here....and separated from our children. Any weekend and all holidays are difficult to handle, they seem to magnify the impact of the long range separation for her. Karen is tough. She's a survivor. Her number one fan in admiration is ME.

10:15 P.M. — Karen moved the rest of our stuff into the new apartment and cleaned while she was there. Wore her out. Holidays also seem to bring an air of depression to the hospital. Can't explain it but the gloom sometimes hangs in the air as dense as a rain cloud. Even the nurses and doctors appear to sense this invisible "holiday" cloud. We talked to the rest of our kids this afternoon. Ricky sounded good and was making last minute preparations for his Washington, D.C. trip. Naturally, his mom knew he couldn't possibly pack without her help, so she offered assistance over the phone. I think Ricky will be glad to get on the road. Karen caught Melissa and Cheryl between sunbathing and boy watching at their Grandma Rockman's in Florida. Sounded like they were having the time of their lives. Both were sunburned already. We had cautioned them about the Florida sun but being teenagers, they already seemed to know everything they needed to know about EVERYTHING. Then I recalled how smart I was when I was their age and decided to save my breath [and Karen's] without any further ado. Melissa was worried about me [distorted rumors were circulating among her friends] until Karen put her mind at ease. The kids all sounded fine and that knowledge made us feel secure. Our phone has rang off the hook all day long. Family and friends calling to make sure that we know we haven't been forgotten. We're ready to call it quits for tonight. Am going to try to read and unwind. Am whipped, but I actually dread the thought of trying to sleep. Too much to emotionally contend with when the lights go out! Please God, help me get some rest and deliver me from the barrage of depressing thoughts that plague me each night.

•DAY 21: MONDAY, MARCH 27, 1989 — 7:20 A.M.

Pain remains all the way across my abdomen. Really drives me to think. And not always good thoughts, I must admit. Positive, positive, positive, trying to maintain a positive attitude. Karen says she can tell I'm agitated this morning. Probably am. Had another restless night with more time spent gazing at the ceiling and dwelling on ugly thoughts. Had recurring nightmare about cancer spreading to my lymph nodes, contaminating the lymph node system all the way to below my collarbones. It was so vivid that when I awoke I really was not sure that it was a dream. Frightens me terribly when I wake and feel the panic this nightmare breeds rushing through my whole body. Took a few minutes to reassure myself logically that it was JUST a bad dream. Each time it occurs I have to regroup and start all over with positive thoughts and actions. I refuse to let cancer bully my conscious mind like it dominates my unconscious mind. On days which begin like this particular one it takes an almost superhuman effort.

6:30 P.M. — Supposed to start my 2nd course of chemo tomorrow but Logo informed us that my counts are still low in some areas. One of those areas is neutrophils, which are white blood cells that come from vertebrae blood and help make up our body's immune system. My count for neutrophils was 900 when they drew blood early this a.m. The count must be at least 1500 before Logo will start the next course. This is a downer because it is VERY important to me that I start each session 21 days apart. Basic reasoning. If I don't begin treatment on schedule, it keeps us in Texas longer and away from our family that much longer. Each and every night I try to remember to pray, "Please Lord, no delays and no complications." My appetite is not back to normal yet. Am forcing down half portions just so the doctors don't put me back on intravenous feeding. Took a l-o-n-g-g-g walk today. Karen went to our apartment to wash clothes, arrange the furniture and pickup our mail before noon. I got the brilliant idea to walk there, catch Karen and ride the shuttle bus back to the hospital with her. Great idea...but poor planning! The walk to our apartment was over two miles and I got lost. To make a long story short, I missed connecting with Karen at the apartment and had to call a cab to return to the hospital. Ended up with huge blisters on my right foot. Blisters, and any other open sores, can be dangerous during chemotherapy. Karen gave me a chewing out and at this point I do not have any long [walking] trips planned for the near future. Still "thinking shrink." Until tomorrow...Goodnight.

Chapter 7

VB IV:

SECOND COURSE
of CHEMOTHERAPY

This course of chemotherapy consists of two drugs administered back to back for five straight days [24-hour periods]. The drugs are called vinblastine and bleomycin. They are given intravenously in a staggered sequence. This is similar to the administration of my 1st course of chemo. Specifically, during this course of chemotherapy I will start with vinblastine, when that dose is finished the med nurses will hang [suspend from I.V. pole] the bleomycin, and when that dose is completed it's back to the vinblastine.

This process of one drug and then the other will be repeated nonstop for the five day period. Believe me, as I stated earlier, these are radical amounts of chemo drugs over a continuous five day period. Remember also, my courses of treatment are scheduled for 21 day intervals. The 21 days are figured like a woman's menstrual cycle. For instance, if I were to start a session of chemotherapy on April 1st the next session would then be scheduled to start on April 22nd. Exactly 21 days apart. As you can see, the 21 day cycle INCLUDES the five days the drugs are administered and only leaves 16 days [after the drugs are infused] to allow your blood counts to return to any degree of normalcy. This is a very tight regimen. With sessions this close your body does not have time to fully recover from the effects of the chemo drugs before it is time to start the next session of chemotherapy. The schedule is tight but necessary when fighting my type of cancer. The cells that make up the malignant tumor need to be bombarded with the chemo BEFORE they can build up a resistance to the chemo drug and its neutralizing effect. This is one more lesson the medical profession apparently learned the hard way.

Prior to taking you back into the daily journal format for this 2nd course of chemo, I should share information learned from the 1st course. Mistakenly, I had believed that when the drugs for each session were finished being administered, the side effects would also cease. That is NOT how it works. Some symptoms of side effects hit me immediately and some came on gradually. In a delayed reaction,other side effects surfaced and came on days after the chemo was administered but are still with me. Such as the terrible stomach cramps and hellatious earaches. In the other extreme were the side effects that came on hard, did their damage and then disappeared. For example: the cisplatin episode I vividly described in *Chapter Six* is painfully etched in my memory. But, one redeeming point concerning the side effects of cisplatin is that there was an end in sight. When I receive cisplatin next time around I now understand that I'll be very sick and nauseated for about 24 hours and then require a few more days to recover my strength. The side effects are severe, yet short-lived. Therefore, for me personally, with a drug like cisplatin the end justifies the means.

In my opinion, the slower hitting side effects are much worse to deal with because it appears they hold on longer, breaking down the patients body over a sustained period of time. When considering the effects of chemotherapy, about the only thing you can be relatively certain of is that you WILL HAVE some kind of side effects while taking these drugs. What those side effects will be, when they will begin and how long they will last is not predictable. Each patient's tolerance and susceptibility is uniquely their own.

JOURNAL ENTRIES
• *DAY 22: TUESDAY, MARCH 28, 1989 — 11:30 A.M.*
The day is only half done but has been quite busy with

volunteer visitors, doctors' rounds and phone calls. Two friends from Michigan called before 7:00 a.m. We talked shop and horses. Shop, as in my old business; and horses, as in trotters and pacers [racehorses]. Good to hear from both "Bills." Our floor has lost two patients to death in the last week. I knew the latest cancer victim quite well. Logo told us this morning, during his rounds, that Patrick "B" had died last night. He had the room right next to mine before he was rushed to Intensive Care [ICU] last Saturday. Patrick was mentioned previously because I had visited with him a few times. Even though I was aware that he wasn't doing real well it still came as a genuine shock to hear about his death. He was a quiet, trusting young man. At 25 years old, he was just a kid. Patrick died from testicular non-seminoma cancer that had metastasized to his brain and spine. Did not escape my notice that Patrick succumbed to the same type of cancer with which I have been diagnosed. Scary. Very scary.

6:45 P.M. — Logo called the 9th floor nursing station and had them tell me that my counts were still down and I would not be starting my next treatment until they came back up. The delay hurts. I realize that the decision to delay treatment is to protect me but it is still a downer. I'm ready mentally. I want [and need] to get started so I can get out of here on schedule [my schedule that is]. Status report: cramps, cramps and more cramps; eyes burning; rash on my neck; and last but not least, my head hair is almost gone. Non-existent might be a more accurate description. I keep smiling and carry all the pain inside. Karen senses I'm hurting and is always there to lean on. Her devotion to OUR cause is evident hour to hour and day by day. That supreme patience she possesses helps keep her emotionally together. Wish I could borrow some of that patience! Am not relishing the opportunity to sleep tonight. If tonight's quest for sleep follows the usual pattern I'll probably wrestle with my own thoughts for a good portion of the night. Seems to go with the territory. Will be praying that I start my next treatment tomorrow.

•*DAY 23: WEDNESDAY, MARCH 29, 1989 — 12:15 P.M.*
Took a long walk outside this morning. Laid down on the

concourse grass in front of the Anderson complex and did some heavy meditating. That's where Karen found me to tell me my counts were up enough to start the 2nd course of chemo. The neutrophil count had risen from 1050 to 1800 in the last 21 hours. A jump of this magnitude is unusual to say the least. This white blood cell count [neutrophils] is what had been holding up my treatment. You never saw anyone so happy to take chemotherapy. Despite knowing I was going to be miserable, I was ecstatic to begin and get back *on schedule.* For the doctors, schedule means a set timetable for treatment. For me, schedule means countdown to going home. Thanks God, for hearing my request to get this treatment going.

4:50 P.M. — Just began my 2nd session of chemo. Have been receiving vinblastine through the I.V. pump for about 20 minutes and have a headache now to accompany my ever present cramps. Vinblastine is also recognized by the name of velban. This drug is known for a number of distinct side effects. Primary on the list is muscle aches. In addition, it can cause infection and bowel paralysis. Also on the list of potential side effects is mouth sores, heart inflammation and you guessed it, headaches. All in all, sounds like some nasty stuff, doesn't it? With no complications the dispensing of this course of chemo should be finishing up on Monday, April 3rd, sometime in the late afternoon. Listen to me, just started the treatment and I'm already charting when I'll be finished. Admittedly, my impatience is poorly disguised. Karen and I have been discussing sending her back home for a few days. We haven't made a decision yet but are considering some specific dates after this session of chemo is completed. We have some problems at home to iron out. Should mention that a number of well-meaning individuals have sent us books and even tapes with EVERY viable approach there is in battling cancer. We cannot possibly read them all, but we are trying to peruse most of them. They represent love, care and concern so we are sincerely grateful for the effort. Worries over our kids are weighing heavy on both our minds today. Some days are worse than others, again, especially for Karen. She knows about where they should be and what they should be doing every hour of the day. The kids and their demanding schedules were her daily life. Hence, the routine is indelibly imprinted in her mind. I can see that faraway look come into her eyes often during the course of a day and sense that she is wondering about the kids' whereabouts and welfare at that precise moment. She tries to suppress it but the anguish on her face cannot be hidden. It hurts me to know I'm indirectly responsible for this separation. We are going to take a walk before Karen eats dinner. This will give us a chance to talk and regroup.

•DAY 24: THURSDAY, MARCH 30, 1989 — 7:10 A.M.

Had a rough night. Neither Karen nor myself slept good. My muscles ache all over and I continue to have chills and diarrhea. My body hurts as if it's the day after an auto accident or the first day of football practice. At least four times a day I'm gargling sodium bicarbonate, baking soda in laymen terms, in conjunction with coating [swishing] the inside of my mouth with Milk of Magnesia. This routine is to prevent mouth sores and oral infection. My mother-in-law is an R.N. [Registered Nurse] and she put me on to the Milk of Mag trick. Seems to work. I've had the misfortune of witnessing other patients with mouth sore side effects and they were totally miserable. It qualifies as a complication to me and I am determined to avoid ANYTHING which can hinder or halt chemo treatment. Any delay is contrary to my goal of ridding my body completely of cancer and returning home as soon as possible.

1:20 P.M. — Dr. James Cox just stopped by our room to visit for a few minutes. Karen asked him a general question about my eventual surgery and he relieved her concerns immediately. Dr. Cox promised again to bring his wife with him the next time he dropped into our room. His wife is a doctor at M.D. Anderson and therefore has a busy schedule herself. Learned a new name for muscle pain...it's called myalgia. See, chemotherapy is good for something. It will broaden your vocabulary and allow you to show off in front of the other patients and spouses by brandishing your newly discovered medical terms. With vinblastine being pumped into my veins I'm sure I'll be using the term "myalgia" in future conversations. Doctors are still trying to take one of my testicles. They feel that one of them is the primary site which emitted the tumor in my abdomen and back. I keep telling them that I've grown quite attached to my testicles [literally] over the years and would like to keep BOTH of them. I'm attempting to be facetious and witty but the truth is that removing a testicle bothers me for more reasons than one. First off, the doctors are not absolutely certain that I have testicular non-seminoma. I'm being treated for the mixed-cell variety of non-seminoma but that is what leaves the doubt. A mixed-cell tumor shows a mixture of different types of malignant cells. One of those cells obviously indicates a close similarity to the cancerous tumor identified as sarcoma because that's what I was originally diagnosed as having. Both in Michigan and here, in Texas. Too much uncertainty for me to be comfortable with any decision to surgically remove a testicle. Second off, even with the doctors and now the pathology department leaning towards mixed cell non-seminoma, they are not sure WHICH testicle is the culprit, if indeed, either one is the primary site. Personally, I don't want EITHER testicle removed much less the wrong testicle. Logo says we will discuss it down the road, he warns that I better concentrate on the life-threatening tumor in my abdomen right now. Easy for him to say, I'm the one that could end up neutered down the road! I relayed all this latest information to my brother, Craig, then told him if he calls and I'm speaking in a high-pitched voice, he'll know what happened. We laughed but each of us knew that I was worried about this eventual decision. Karen keeps reminding me, "One day at a time, Rick, one day at a time." I hate it when she patronizes me, but I love her and realize she's right.

10:15 P.M. — This concludes another day in the life. It's now tumor shrinking time. For the last few days, when I take my daily shower I mentally envision that the water spraying my body is a cleansing elixir which is blessed by God and dissolving the tumor in me. This kind of creative imaging helps combat the worry of metastasizing and at the same time keeps my mind active with positive ideas. The fact that the shower water touches all parts of my body lets me visualize that I'm preventing the tumor from spreading. I continue to have these horrible dreams [nightmares would be more appropriate] concerning cancer spreading to the lymph nodes below my collarbones. Watching the misfortunes of other patients, I've inadvertently discovered that uncontrollable metastazation is an eventual death sentence. It's scary but I continue to speak positive and contend with this information only in my mind. Anyway, these mental imagery exercises seem to help. They make me feel I'm assisting my own cause by refusing to lay here in a semi-catatonic state and give in to the always ugly, sometimes terminal thoughts. Almost forgot, they hung the 2nd drug of this VB4 treatment, which is bleomycin, at 5:00 p.m. Update on kids: Ricky should be getting home from his class trip to Washington, D.C. before midnight [Michigan time]. Stacey and Randy came home from their Grandma Ouellette's yesterday. Melissa and Cheryl are still in Florida winding up their Easter vacation. Will call tomorrow and find out how they all fared. Goodnight and pleasant dreams.

•DAY 25: FRIDAY, MARCH 31, 1989 — 7:35 A.M.
Time flies when you're having fun! This is the line I greeted Karen with when we awoke. Actually, we both had a restless night but she did break a smile with my obnoxious attempt at a little humor. Karen tossed and turned much of the night and I was up and down to the bathroom often. The bathroom visits come as no surprise with the amount of drugs they are pumping through my I.V. lines. Am extremely thirsty since starting this treatment. Has to be the chemo. Can't seem to drink enough fluids to satisfy my body's need or my own thirst. Pain in my stomach from the cramps woke me out of a sound sleep twice during the night. Sleep does not come easy after these cramping bouts. Cramps and headache remain with me but the earache is gone this morning. If you can believe this, the scalp of my head has been irritated and sore for two straight days. It's like my skin aches. Probably sounds weird but that describes the pain. Can't be from sunburn since I've been wearing a hat for my outdoor walks. So, it must be an unusual side effect from the vinblastine or bleomycin I'm receiving.

8:45 P.M. — My friend and fellow patient Kevin "M" is sick today. Mouth sores have set in and his neutrophil count is 0. Not good because the neutrophil count indicates he has no white blood cells with which to fight off infection or fever. His tongue is so swollen he can hardly speak. An older man, across the corridor and on the other side of our floor looks like he is in a very bad way. The man's name is Victor "S." We had talked briefly 2 or 3 times in the past week but when I went to his room this afternoon he was heavily sedated. Met his wife, Mary, and she informed me that she's aware her husband is dying. She feels that in a way, it is a blessing because he's suffered so terribly much as they have battled with cancer over the past year. This woman is a tender sweetheart and yet, tough as nails. During one of our earlier conversations Victor related that the doctors were never quite sure where the cancer originated but that it had spread slowly and relentlessly for the last months. He also told me that he's refused any further chemotherapy or radiation treatment. I hope he has a restful night. Enough words about sick people. Stacey and Randy brightened our day by sending us three cards apiece and a box of goodies to share. Their cards and enclosed notes were real "tear jerkers." They took the edge off a rough day.

•DAY 26: SATURDAY, APRIL 1, 1989 — 12:00 NOON

Karen has been occupying herself for the biggest part of the morning with a jigsaw puzzle that my sister, Debbie, sent via the mail. It's a tough one according to Karen but I'm sure she is up to the challenge with that mountain of patience she possesses. Walked for over an hour outside on the cement concourse. Very hot and humid. Went to see Kevin when I returned and discovered he continues to have a rough road to travel. The mouth sores have spread down into his throat. He can barely swallow and breathes only through his nose. Man, do I feel for him and man, am I gargling and coating my mouth with Milk of Magnesia so I don't contract those mouth sores. Makes me miserable just looking at Kevin. Chatted with Victor "S's" wife for 15 minutes. Mary told me that Victor has had some lucid moments where they converse but not very many recently. She is at his bedside all day, every day. Next to Victor and Kevin's condition, my cramps, muscle aches and other assorted side effects don't seem nearly as bad. Like my dad always said as we were growing up, "Just look around, there's ALWAYS someone worse off than you."

10:05 P.M. — Logo was in this afternoon. Passed on the good word that my AFP is still dropping. At present it is down to 120. He took time to explain that it needs to be under 5 before it is considered medically neutralized. Logo also stated that the count must be under 5 and stable before surgery to remove the tumor will be scheduled. From this point, he went on to say that bleomycin breaks down and destroys muscle tissue and is most likely the reason I have so much pain in my neck and arms. Myalgia, which means muscle aches [remember?], does not do justice to some of the pain spasms I've been enduring. Without exaggerating, every joint in my body seems to ache. Along the lines of thinking positive I count my blessings that I have so far dodged any mouth sores or infections. But, counting my blessings does not belie the fact that vinblastine and bleomycin are some very nasty stuff. Let's call it a day on that note and get into the mental imagery of shrinking the tumor.

•DAY 27: SUNDAY, APRIL 2 1989 — 11:20 A.M.
Been a dreary day so far. The sun has not shown itself yet. Could smell the threat of rain in the air as I took my morning stroll around the complex. Did two laps around and had to push myself to do that much. No energy and same side effects nagging my body. My thirst seems unquenchable. I try to keep moving and talk positive even on these days that are naturally gloomy. It remains an effort. We are still trying to get Karen home to Michigan in the very near future. We've tentatively decided on this coming Friday, April 7th, to fly her home. Karen was worried about my welfare while she would be gone so I asked Logo to intervene and reassure her. He shot down Karen's objections by casually reminding her that what happens will happen, whether she is present or not. Logo said you can't plan it, you just go home when it feels right. He concluded by convincing Karen that there are no critical

decisions to be made at this time.

3:50 P.M. — Met two more patients today. Dwight "P" is on our floor and being treated for bladder cancer. Right now his chemo treatments are halted because he's experiencing stomach complications. Similar to my earlier situation, the doctors are discussing surgery for Dwight if the stomach inflammation does not calm down. The other patient is a fellow Michigander. His name is Larry "G" and his wife's name is Bernadette. They're from Hemlock, Michigan and that is only 55-65 miles from our fair city of Fenton. Larry has renal cell carcinoma. He already had one kidney removed three years ago due to the renal cell cancer. Was great visiting with folks from our home state. Nice people. Karen and I would have enjoyed meeting them under better circumstances. Kevin "M" continues to fight the side effects of his last treatment, which was VB4, the same one I'm taking right now. He finished that session ten days ago but has been hit hard by mouth and throat sores. Kevin's white blood cells remain extremely low and his neutrophil count reflects this fact. Victor "S" continues to hang on and is receiving heavy doses of pain medication.

8:50 P.M. — Must be family night. All of my brothers and sisters have called to say "hi" and Karen's mom and dad, plus her brother Dean phoned. Later, my mom and dad called to check on us. Difficult for me to talk this evening. My ears are ringing, head and both sides of my jaw ache. The jaw pain is a new discomfort and so is the chemical taste in my mouth which I noticed this morning. The chemical taste has gotten steadily stronger all day. The odor is terrible. It smells like I've been gargling with iodine and tastes the same as it smells. Feel worn out but not sleepy. Am going outside and walk. My walks are a self-reckoning time for me. They allow me the private time to get back on a positive train of thought if I've slipped into doubt or self-pity during the course of a day. Despite the intense effort it often takes to just get out of the hospital bed, my walking excursions are rejuvenating to mind and body. It's been swell! More entries tomorrow.

•DAY 28: MONDAY, APRIL 3, 1989 — 10:35 A.M.
Karen's gone to the apartment to do our laundry and pick up mail. She's got to be back before noon because a couple of lady volunteers from the Presbyterian church are taking her out for lunch. A lunch surrounded by healthy people for a change will be great medicine for her mental outlook. Just what the doctor ordered! Karen befriended a lady named Kathy "G" at breakfast. She is the mother of a young patient on our floor. Kathy said her son, Peter, is experiencing some severe side effects from chemo but would love some company. I wandered down to his room a little while ago and introduced myself. Surprisingly, he is another testicular non-seminoma patient. With that common ground we compared notes and chatted for a few minutes. All I can say is that Peter has had quite a struggle already and doesn't look to be out of harm's way yet. Peter and his mother are from Houston and their residence is less than five miles from the M.D. Anderson facility. Today is the last day of my 2nd session. Should be finished receiving the vinblastine and bleomycin about 5:00 p.m.

10:10 P.M. — Here's one for the record books. I have a bunch of peach fuzz trying to grow back on my head. Logo jokingly said at lunch time that I'm supposed to lose my hair, NOT grow new hair. Had become accustomed to looking at myself with a bald head for the last week so this was quite a surprise when baby-fine hair sprouted over night. Logo says to enjoy it 'cuz it won't last long. Another day is winding down and that puts us one day closer to home. Am not going to list my usual rash of side effects. Suffice to say that I continue to experience basically the same ones. Reading my journal entries one would guess that I walk around complaining all day, every day. Not so! I speak positive or don't speak at all. Karen Marie is the only person who sees me with my guard down and starting to feel sorry for myself. When it happens, I usually take one of my rehabilitative "loner" walks to get back on track. Apparently, writing down some of the negative thoughts and occurrences that come our way during a typical day in the hospital helps get the depressing venom out of my system. Besides, there seems to be a fine line between talking a lie and living the truth. I record how I actually feel and act how I'd like to feel. At any rate, I firmly believe that scribbling my journal entries helps me cope on a day to day basis. Whatever it takes I will do to defeat cancer! Finished 2nd session at 6:20 p.m. Two courses down and only three or four to go...I hope.

•DAY 29: TUESDAY, APRIL 4, 1989 — 5:10 P.M.

Met another patient on our floor who is being treated for the same cancer I am. His name is Carl "M" and he comes from a small town near St. Louis, Missouri. I had seen Carl at one of the testing areas over a week ago but did not have any communication with him. I did hear parts of his cancer story as he conveyed it to another patient waiting for his respective C.A.T. scan. It didn't sound good then as I picked up pieces of the conversation and it sounds even worse now that I've heard the whole tale. Eighteen months ago, Carl had a large tumor surgically removed at a hospital in St. Louis. No follow-up treatment [radiation, chemo, etc.] was ordered by his doctors. When he returned for a routine check-up his blood markers [AFP count, remember?] indicated that cancer was somewhere in his body again. He was informed that the doctors in St. Louis could do no more for him and that's how he ended up at M.D. Anderson in Houston. He has had chemotherapy and radiation while here in Houston and his blood markers are still elevated which indicates cancer cells remain somewhere in his body. This is the scenario that every cancer patient lives to dread...the fear of reoccurrence. Carl's story gets me down. Seems like all I hear are horror stories of tumors, spreading and reoccurrence. I keep telling myself that I'm different — and in the same breath, PRAY that I am. "Different" here, from what I can see, is to be cured and beat cancer. Took a walk outside in the warm Texas sun to get my head back on straight. Walked for over an hour working on attitude adjustment as me and God had a heart-to-heart talk. Told God that I wasn't better than anyone else BUT I did expect a DIFFERENT outcome than the vast majority of ones which I was witnessing. Sounds kind of contradictory now, as

I record our private conversation, but I rationalize the effort with the solemn oath that I steadfastly REFUSE to give in to cancer.

9:05 P.M. — Asked for some pain medication to take the edge off the cramps and muscle pain. Kevin "M" is up and moving around. He does not feel good but realizes that he needs to push himself or he'll be sick even longer with the side effects he's encountering. Trying to get letters written to all of our kids so K.M. can take them with her when she goes home this coming Friday. Hope the letters dissolve some of the difficulties we are having with the kids. Karen intends to iron some of these rough spots out when she gets home. Been another up and down day. It's like a roller coaster ride with more downs than ups. Logo ordered intravenous pain medication to get me through the night. Hope it helps because I feel "wired" with pain right now. Tomorrow can only be better. Think shrink and pleasant dreams.

•DAY 30: WEDNESDAY, APRIL 5 1989 — 8:00 A.M.
Another restless night for us. Karen fretted about going home and leaving me alone while I itched and worried myself awake. She thinks I must be allergic to the pain medication I received intravenously because I spent most of the night itching at my face and arms. Asked the nurses what all the commotion was at 10:00 p.m. last night and they related that Victor "S" had died. We were very sorry to hear this, especially for his wife, Mary. Victor had suffered a long time and it was probably a blessing for him to die in his sleep as he did. He was in his late 50's as far as age. At least, I think that is what the nurses said. Relatively speaking, he was young regardless of his exact age. I view it as another decent human being lost to this monster called cancer. We are all going to die someday, but I keep asking myself, "Do we have to die sick and bed ridden?" I never gave too much thought to sickness and death until I arrived here. Now, it's a daily battle NOT to think about sickness and death. This is one of those days where you could cut the cloud of oppression in the air with a knife.

7:35 P.M. — Karen is down calling her mom on the AT&T free phone. Yes, you read correctly. That's free as in REALLY

FREE, no strings attached. No charge for one phone call per day to anywhere in the world. Yes, you read that correctly also. My understanding of the service is that you can call ANYWHERE in the world for 10 minutes if you are a patient or spouse at the M.D. Anderson Cancer Clinic. AT&T donated this special perk to a select few hospitals in the U.S.A. for one full year. Many patients at M.D. Anderson are from another country so this is a chance for them to call home and speak to loved ones at no charge. Not to mention the patients who use the service to call within the continental United States. It's a beautiful gesture from big business and AT&T deserves some accolades. The pattern of becoming sicker in the late afternoon and early evening is still a daily occurrence. There's apparently no viable explanation. Cramps and rest of the usual side effects are still with me. The terrible mouth taste remains and Karen says my skin is even giving off an odor from the effects of vinblastine and bleomycin. Have to keep busy and get through the next 4-5 days and then the symptoms should let up. Taking dilaudid in pill form for pain medication. Very tired after last night's itching bout. Both of us will be trying to hit the sack early tonight. We'll call the kids tomorrow probably. Karen just snapped a picture of me and our luxury accommodations. I think she enjoys me being bald-headed even though she maintains that the snapshots are to cherish a year from now when all of this is behind us and we can't recall how forlorn we looked and felt. Now that's positive attitude.

•DAY 31: THURSDAY, APRIL 6, 1989 — 8:20 A.M.
Went for a long walk at 2:15 a.m. Muscle aches and severe cramping in my stomach had awakened me from a sound sleep. Traipsed around the concourse outside and enjoyed the warm Houston breeze as I tried to relax the pain into subsiding. Quiet and peaceful during these early morning hours. Houstonites driving by in their cars stared but I'm well past the point of getting a complex. Don't blame the motorists anyway. I'd probably stare too if I saw some nut pulling an I.V. stand and pump around at 2:00 in the morning. At any rate, the late night and early morning jaunts are sanity time

for me. The panic I sometimes feel is quelled by these peaceful excursions. It's a time when I always reflect on the fact that this is a personal battle between me and cancer. With medicine, logic and surgery offering no guarantees, God is the ally I lean on during these private walks. It helps to think I have a mentor with more control over this cancer disease than I have — namely, an omniscient God.

1:05 P.M. — Karen is starting to gather items for her trip home tomorrow. Any reservations or guilt she was dealing with are giving way to excitement at the prospect of seeing all of our children. She needs to get away and the trip home will be good for her and all the kids. Karen also will be confronting some minor dilemmas on the home front so it is not all fun and games that she's going home to. Despite the potential problems she is still excited.

3:45 P.M. — Kevin "M" went home to Corpus Christi [Texas] today. He certainly did not look well but said he was ready to get out of here. Think the hospital environment was wearing on him and his emotions. Needed the security and seclusion of his own home. Even though it's a three hour drive from Houston to Corpus Christi for Kevin, we are still envious because at least he is truly going HOME. Karen dragged me to the apartment on a four hour pass today. She wanted to pack for the trip home and just plain get me away from the hospital. When we returned, Karen's Uncle Bob and Aunt Waneta were standing at the entrance to the 1st floor elevators. A pleasant surprise. We exchanged greetings and from there Karen went off and visited with them as I headed for the 9th floor to grab some rest. They took Karen to dinner and she really enjoyed their company. As recent retirees, Bob and Waneta were touring the Southwestern United States and had stopped especially to see Karen on the Western leg of the trip. The afternoon symptoms are starting to surface. My stomach is really acting up. Some of the cramps grab me to the point where I double over until the pain eases. Phone is ringing, that's my cue to cut this entry short. Still thinking shrink and trying to MAKE it happen.

•DAY 32: FRIDAY, APRIL 7, 1989 — 7:05 A.M.
Karen Marie flies out in four hours, she leaves M.D. Anderson
for Houston Hobby Airport in about two hours. She is having
mixed emotions this morning but I expected this late reaction.
I told her one last time that I would be fine and not to worry
about me because she would have plenty to fret about at
home. That seemed to appease her conscience. Will miss her
terribly, she has spoiled me with her attention and devotion.
Did not get much sleep last night but I do feel better today.
Jaw pain, head and ear aches have let up considerably. My
arms, neck and shoulders do not ache like they have for the
past 8-9 days either.
11:40 A.M. — Karen departed for the airport at 9:30 a.m. Her
Northwest Airlines flight should be airborne right about now.
Kathy "G" volunteered to drive her there. Her son, Peter, is
the young man having so many severe side effects from
chemotherapy. One of his side effects was a spot that he
itched on the left side of his face that became an open sore and
turned into a huge, infected boil. It is scabbing over now but
at one time this lesion covered the whole left side of his face.
This is a prime example of the type of complications I am
trying to avoid. This particular side effect delayed Peter's next
chemo treatment for almost three weeks. If you recall, he is
being treated for testicular non-seminoma cancer. Karen had
planned to take a shuttle to the airport but Kathy very
graciously insisted on driving her. We appreciated the gesture. Dropped into a patient's room this morning that has
been here [off and on] for a long time. His name is Sid "P." He
was friendly but not much of a talker as he waited for his wife
to return with some good ol' junk food. Told him I'd stop by
again or he could drop into my room for a visit.
7:35 P.M. — I miss Karen Marie already. Like I said, she spoils
me with her love and attention and it is easy to take for
granted until she's absent. Spend much time roaming the
halls and snooping on different hospital floors. My nomadic
wanderings are enlightening but also sobering. Have seen
some sad, sad cases up on the 10th floor and visited with
relatives of sad cases in the Intensive Care waiting room. The
phone has been very busy. Karen would normally answer it

but with her absent the duty is mine alone. Each time it rings I have another reminder that she is absent. I continue to pray each night for this huge tumor in my abdomen to shrink. Have added to the list my concerns about a primary tumor site. For the last week or so, I've prayed for God to undeniably confirm this site. In other words, if one of my testicles is cancerous I've prayed to know for sure which one. Well, decided as I was walking this afternoon to quit asking God to be a substitute doctor. I have revamped my prayers and reminded God that *He can do anything*. With that premise in mind, I've done some heavy duty praying that there is *NO PRIMARY SITE*. Once you admit you are scared, it's relatively easy to ask for faith and strength in God's name. I feel like a hypocrite sometimes when I call on this God that I've chosen to pretty much neglect over the past years. I ask anyway. Don't know anyone or anything else to give me the assurance I'm looking for to beat this cancer. Can't wait for Karen to call from home. Dying to hear how the homecoming reception went. Whoops! Must remind myself to stop using that term. Poor choice of words in my predicament. Once again, until tomorrow think shrink AND *no* primary tumor site.

•DAY 33: SATURDAY, APRIL 8, 1989 — 6:20 A.M.

It's abnormally quiet this morning. Even the nurses are moving about quietly. Not accustomed to getting up without Karen present. Probably will even miss her taking the customary 45-50 minutes in the bathroom with which she ceremoniously begins each day. We are definitely creatures of habit. Karen finally called at 9:30 p.m. last evening. Lisa and Rick [my sister and our brother-in-law] plus all the kids surprised her at the airport. Karen received five weeks worth of hugs and kisses before they left the terminal. She loved it. *11:15 P.M.* — Rode the exercise bike [carefully, I might add] and took my walks off and on throughout the day. Ran into a patient I have not mentioned yet that I had met at Station #10 a good month ago. I call him "crazy Mel." That first time I met him he told me his whole cancer story in less than five minutes. In a nutshell, Mel has an incurable form of lymphoma. On top of that the cancer has metastasized and gone to his brain. The medical staff at M.D. Anderson had informed him the day we met that his only remaining option was to try experimental chemo drugs that were still unproven. What's amazing to me was his "that's the way it goes" attitude in response to this news. When we bumped into each other today he said he was taking some of those experimental drugs and if they didn't work to control his cancer there was nothing else available. Mel didn't complain but said some of the side effects he was experiencing were "kick-ass." While telling me this he never blinked an eye. Reminded me again of the first time we met when he ended our cancer conversation by inviting me to go to some topless bar on the outskirts of Houston. He shifted from speaking about impending death to partying without a pause. This time he wanted me to go smoke some reefer in the hospital parking ramp. When I declined, he offered to set up a standing chess match each morning at 10:00 a.m. in the hospital lobby. From strippers to marijuana to chess...Mel's mind and mouth moved too fast for me to keep up with him. He switched channels in a conversation before you could draw a deep breath. Maybe you can understand why I took the liberty of nicknaming him "crazy Mel." His antics and invitations were funny but also sadly transparent. As Mel strolled away with his back to me I sensed that he realized his days on this earth were winding down. Mel was trying to shove as many "good times" as he could into these last weeks or months of his life. Another sad case of cancer strikes again! Think shrink and say a prayer for Mel.

•DAY 34: SUNDAY, APRIL 9, 1989 — 10:40 A.M.

Woke up and looked around for Karen Marie. Hard habit to break. Miss her immensely. Called Karen's mom and suggested that Karen needed her at our house for moral support while she was home for these few days. Helen said she was way ahead of me and was driving down to Fenton right after church this morning. We small talked for a couple more minutes and then I let her go. Puts my mind at ease knowing that Helen can be there for Karen. Sid "P", a guy I met three days back, ducked his head into my room and we shot the breeze for a few minutes. I think he said he'd been in the Intensive Care Unit. Hard to believe he's up and moving around. Sid was walking very slow and seemed overly tired. To be downright honest he looked terrible. Can only hope the man feels better than he appeared.

9:45 P.M. — Eddie "T" is back on the floor for another chemo session. Eddie says his last C.A.T. scan indicated the tumor under his right rib cage is shrinking. This was excellent news and I was glad for him. He still has not lost his head hair. Supposedly, one cannot equate hair loss with success or failure of the treatment. The fact remains that Eddie is the only patient I know who has not lost his hair yet to chemo. Emphasizes once again that everyone is truly different. Had a minor mishap with my I.V. line this evening. The suture site for my CVC line had some tape on it that was irritating my arm so one of the nurses attempted to remove the tape. She accidentally snipped the line where it enters into my arm with scissors. Blood shot all over until I grabbed what was left of the I.V. line and crimped it off. The nurse felt terrible. She put in a call for the Infusion Therapy team and they were able to repair the line without implanting a new CVC line. The situation presented a couple of scary moments but all's well that ends well. Left side of my tongue is swollen and bleeding a little. Mouth sores are trying to set in and I'm trying to prevent them from getting a foothold. Cramps and muscle pain are constant. Other than these "small" aches and pains I feel good. Am headed outside for an evening stroll with my good friend, Mr. I.V. Pole. Tomorrow will be a better day. Goodnight and sweet dreams.

•DAY 35: MONDAY, APRIL 9, 1989 — 7:55 A.M.
My brother Glenn is slipping into town to see me sometime today. Don't know what time his flight is arriving from Detroit so I plan to sit tight until he gets here. Looking forward to seeing him. Had spells of sweating to go along with the usual abdomen pain last night. Soaked my bed sheets with perspiration. Some nights I have chills and some nights I have sweating. Never know which...or why. It's raining outside. Funny how moods seem to be associated

with the weather. Kind of gloomy atmosphere is evident today in the hospital and that reflects what the weather is doing outside. Supposed to clear up before the end of the day. Hope so. BOTH forecasts, inside and outside, should improve if it does. Wondering what the kids and Karen are doing about now. I'm sure Karen is moving in high gear no matter what she is doing. In keeping up with five kids, high gear is about the only speed you're allowed to move.

8:50 P.M. — Glenn arrived at the hospital at 1:30 p.m. He came up to our floor and proceeded to cruise right past me as I stood in the corridor waiting for him. I finally hollered, "Hey, Brother...you looking for me?" We had a good laugh thanks to my baldness and his lack of recognition. I got a four hour pass okayed so we could go to the apartment and I could show Glenn all the ropes. We picked up our mail and then I drove Glenn around demonstrating as much of the area as I had mastered. We headed back to the hospital early. My temp was going up and both of us were tired. Shipped Glenn off to the apartment about twenty minutes ago. He was dead on his feet and wanted to drive while it was still light outside. My temp is 100.4 and my stomach is really acting up. Hurts as bad as it did two nights ago. Along the lines of thinking and talking positive, I know some of this pain will let up; I just don't know exactly when. The pain wears you down after awhile. Never a rest. Am supposed to start another treatment in nine short days. Hoping some of these other side effects disappear by then. For instance, the earaches and headaches. Miss Karen all the time but especially at night. We usually talked a little before turning in each night. It was a pleasant finishing touch to some very unpleasant days. Plan to ride the stationary bike and walk prior to hitting the sack. Until then, thinking shrink and saying prayers for some of my fellow patients who are worse off than yours truly.

•DAY 36: TUESDAY, APRIL 10, 1989 — 9:20 A.M.
Phoned Karen at home about 7:30 a.m. to get a family update before she left the house to run errands. We talked about all of the kids individually. They are coping as well as can be expected. Karen is encountering a couple areas of question-

able behavior concerning the three older kids. We expect them to set a good example for their younger sister and brother. Maybe we expect too much under the circumstances but with our families doing weekly shifts at our house as surrogate parents, good behavior is a must. Our best preventive medicine is to keep the kids occupied and constructively busy. Melissa and Cheryl are holding down part-time jobs after school and weekends. Ricky went to umpire school yesterday. Since he'll be getting paid for Little League umpiring this spring and summer, it qualifies as a job. Stacey and Randy are both involved in extracurricular school activities. Karen is making some tough decisions and setting some unpopular guidelines at home. The stress wears her down but she is handling things as well as they can be handled.

9:50 A.M. — One of my favorite old comedy shows, *I Dream of Jeannie,* was on TV when Logo came by during his morning rounds. Glenn and I were laughing our heads off as I tried to introduce my brother to Dr. Logothetis. Logo said he was glad I felt so good because he was releasing me from the hospital. With a few words of caution about not overdoing it Logo finished by stating that his office would call our apartment and inform me of the readmission date. He ordered a heparin lock for my CVC and said he'd see me again in about a week. Although this declaration took me by surprise, he didn't have to say it twice. After 37 straight days in this hospital room I was ready to go — ANYWHERE! The only bad thing was that I had to pack up all the belongings that we had accumulated over the last five weeks of hospital living. With Glenn's assistance, I packed all our visible items into bags and then went to the hospital pharmacy to fill prescriptions for carafate and dilaudid. One to coat my cramping stomach and the other for pain medication. Glenn carried the bags down to the lobby. From there we were off to the apartment.

6:05 P.M. — By the time we arrived at the apartment the sun was shining and it was a balmy 68 degrees. Glenn and I [mostly Glenn] unloaded the car and toted everything up to our 2nd floor apartment. The phone rang before we were unpacked. Karen would have been proud of me, we only forgot three or four things back at our hospital room. If you recall, I stated that we packed all visible items. Well, am not saying the belongings we missed were invisible but they surely weren't obvious to the human eye. Not to MY eyes at least. The nurses gathered the items I had overlooked, deposited them in a bag and left them at the 9th floor nursing station for me. They then called our apartment phone number to inform us of the oversight. Told them thanks and promised to pick up our belongings tomorrow. Glenn and I decided to go over to the jog path which is a block from our apartment complex. We took a considerably long walk and enjoyed the sunshine as we talked. Gave us the opportunity for a sincere brother to brother conversation. The discussion did us both some good as it disarmed some of Glenn's fears concerning my situation and long range prognosis. At the same time, looking at Glenn was like viewing a caricature of myself [10 years ago] and that reminded me of how I had taken my good health for granted. Youth has a knack for doing that; taking life itself and everyday health for granted. By design, young blood only thinks about living.

8:50 P.M. — Karen called from home earlier tonight. She was actually returning my call from this morning when I phoned to let her know Glenn had arrived and that I had been discharged from the hospital. Missed connecting with her this a.m. because she was shopping with her mom. Upon hearing Karen's voice, could tell immediately that she did not sound like herself. Things apparently were not going too smooth at home. Noticed a lot of tension in her voice during our conversation. Gave Karen an update on my status, discussed the kids and finished our talk by exchanging "I love you's." Before hanging up I asked to say "hello" to her mom. After talking to Helen for a couple minutes I could sense something was definitely wrong on the homefront. Made up my mind then and there that I was going home on the next plane. While talking with Helen, I cupped the phone receiver with my hand and told Glenn what I had in mind. He replied, "If it will make you feel better, go for it, brother." I released my hand from covering the receiver and informed Helen that we would be coming home to Michigan sometime tomorrow. Asked her not to say anything to anyone in case the plans went sour and hung up. Next step was to secure plane tickets as soon as possible. Called Southwest Airlines and reserved two one-way tickets for a noon flight tomorrow from Houston Hobby to Detroit Metro Airport. Southwest Airlines agreed to redeem Glenn's original return ticket for the one-way reservation we had just secured. All systems were go and I was comfortable with the decision. Plain and simple, I felt my presence was needed at home. With tickets out of the way I made plans to catch Dr. Logothetis during his morning rounds and let him know I was headed home but would be back in time to start the next chemotherapy treatment. Been an eventful day and evening so I am signing off. As the British say, "God speed."

•DAY 37: WEDNESDAY, APRIL 12, 1989 — 12:30 P.M.
My brother Glenn and I are on a plane headed home to Michigan. Think it's time to admit again that I am NOT an avid flyer. In fact, the older I get the more difficult it is for me to put my life in the pilot's hands and relax. Frankly, I'm terrible to fly with because each bit of turbulence sends me into reserved panic. Dr. Logothetis wasn't exactly thrilled about my plans to fly home for three days and come back to Houston with Karen on her scheduled return flight. Really did not expect him to understand the urgency but in the end he was gracious regarding my impromptu departure. Logo was worried about my blood counts being low after the last chemo session and making me more susceptible to pick up an infection or virus. Especially, in the close quarters of an airplane. I assured him that I would be alright. He queried with, "Richard, how do you KNOW you will be fine?" My answer was, "Because I have to be." Logo didn't realize it but I was well aware of the risk factor and had spent a good portion of last night praying that I would get through this trip home with NO COMPLICATIONS. Also, had rehashed in my mind that the journey WAS necessary and not just a whim I was satisfying. The conclusion was obvious because here I am; on a flight back to Michigan. Can't wait to see K.M. and all the kids.
11:45 P.M. — It is GREAT to be home. Surprised everyone.

Mostly Karen. She almost went into shock when the kids hollered, "Mom...Dad's home!" She recovered quickly though, after greeting me with a warm kiss and hug, she began an earnest lecture about possible chemo complications and bawled me out with the words, "You shouldn't have come home like this." As with Logo, Karen was worried I would get sick here at home and have no one knowledgeable enough to treat the low blood counts and side effects. Told her not to worry, can't afford to get sick...so I won't. Stacey and Randy were playing baseball with the neighborhood kids when we drove into the driveway. Our yard has always been the neighborhood playground so it did my heart good to see the ritual had not changed during our absence. None of the kids recognized me until I got out of the car. Randy and Stacey kept staring, finally Randy blurted out, "It's Dad!"...as they both ran over to give me a hug. Loved this homecoming. The older kids came straggling home one at a time through the evening and got the surprise of their life when I popped up to greet them. At 166 pounds, bald-headed and weak, I'm quite certain that the kids were taken aback but they disguised their feelings well. It was absolutely fantastic to see all of us together once more. The reality of why I had ventured home settled in when Karen and I went to bed tonight. We discussed the kids and some of the problems we were facing until we were too exhausted to continue. The problems weren't going anywhere so we left it alone until some of these areas of concern could be dealt with. Just seeing our family together again makes me all the more resolute that I have to return healthy and whole for all of them. Concentration! Think shrink!

•DAY 38: THURSDAY, APRIL 13, 1989 — 9:30 A.M.

Beautiful day and great to be back home. Kids all came in and kissed us goodbye before leaving for school. Got a good night's rest and so did Karen. We both needed it badly. Helen, my mother-in-law, gave me two halcion tablets to help sleep and they must have worked. Have a bad headache and heavy-duty stomach cramps this morning. Don't really want anyone to know and have them worrying and asking me questions. Thus, I'll have to suffer quietly and hope they let up soon. My sister Lisa and her husband, Rick, came out this morning to see us. They've been staying at our house and watching our kids for the past few weeks. When Karen came home two days ago it gave them a break in the surrogate parenting role and they returned to THEIR home. For obvious reasons, Lisa and Rick might be the only people happier for me to be home than myself. They've earned a rest. I don't know what Karen and I would do if our family hadn't volunteered to substitute for us in our parenting role at home. Words cannot do justice to our feeling of gratitude. Helen is leaving for home this morning. She's been a wonderful help and steadying influence for Karen. We'll miss her [and her cooking] more than we care to admit when she returns to East Tawas.

6:10 P.M. — Longtime friends of mine came out around lunchtime and visited for awhile. We swapped "war stories" and talked about the good ol' days. Needless to say, our good ol' days conversation did not include sickness, disease or cancer as topics. Most of it centered on golf and "raising hell" in the past. Prior to leaving, Bill and Terry presented us with almost $7200.00 they had collected as a donation from friends in our behalf. We were totally overwhelmed by the generosity of all involved. Karen voiced our feelings best when she said, "We can really use the money and we are SO VERY GRATEFUL. Thanks, from the bottom of our hearts." Have been trying to catch all the kids for a one-on-one talk. Spoke with Ricky last night despite all the confusion my first night home. Caught Cheryl and Randy today for short, but meaningful *tete-a-tetes*. Will try to talk with Melissa and Stacey yet tonight. As far as discipline and behavior, our children all know what is basically expected of them. That does not mean they always behave the way they have been taught. But it does mean they are aware of what is acceptable behavior in our household and what is not. That was the parent side of the talks. The other side was how the kids all seem to feel that we have abandoned them by running off to Houston, Texas. They have a lot of anger pent up and don't seem to comprehend where to direct it. Doesn't take a psychiatrist to understand that their emotions are perfectly natural under the circumstances. I told them each that Mom and I were terribly sorry it had to be this way and that it was just as severe a separation on us as it was on them. Without being dramatic I attempted to convey to each of the kids that we understand their frustration and it is nothing to be ashamed of or carry around guilt over. My approach to the kids was, and will be for the last two, to make them realize the treatment in Texas is to save my life. I informed them that if they wanted Dad around in the future I had to battle cancer and beat it completely. M.D. Anderson Cancer Clinic was the only place we knew of that gave me a chance of doing that. They understood the best they could. At least the problems that we came home to straighten out were being addressed. The kids were having a tough time maintaining respectful attitudes and recognizing figures of authority. Conversely, our children had to accept the rules and personalities of each new set of surrogates that came into our home. The substitute parents had to exert authority, require respect and at the same time be mindful of the unusual circumstances which placed them in our home. Bottom line is that my battle with cancer is TOUGH ON EVERYBODY involved!

8:35 P.M. — Karen and I have been on the run since 6:50 a.m. We have friends and family coming by the house on a steady basis and expect more yet tonight. Have noticed my left leg aching and going numb for the past 2-3 hours. This is a NEW pain. Hope it leaves as suddenly as it came. Until tomorrow, count your blessings...I am.

•DAY 39: FRIDAY, APRIL 14, 1989 — 8:45 A.M.
Thanks to halcion, fatigue and the warm, familiar surroundings of home, Karen and I slept sound again. For myself, two nights in a row of real rest is a new record. Between visitors, found time to talk privately with Melissa and Stacey. Went similar to the discussions I'd had with each of the other kids. Suppressed anger is the best way I can describe the kids' attitude. Told them all, there is nothing shameful about experiencing these hidden emotions. On the contrary, they are perfectly natural. I tried to explain that even though we

understood where they were coming from they would still have to alter and curtail some of their behavior patterns at home. Detailed how selfish and irresponsible attitudes hurt everyone, including them. It just made the situation that much more difficult to endure. Concluded with the words, "Be patient kids, mom and I are going to return home as soon as humanly possible." And I believed those optimistic words. *11:05 P.M.* — The conclusion of another busy, busy day. Karen is completely exhausted. By a rough estimate, we probably had over 35 relatives and friends come by the house to visit and wish us well today. My trip home was a secret initially. Adds credence to the idea that secrets may be the fastest moving and most accurate form of communication in 20th century existence. We enjoyed everyone immensely. Their sincere compassion is like plasma to our eroded emotions and worn out bodies. Karen worked in her "talks" with the kids periodically through the last day and a half. We both feel that we addressed the problem[s] as well as we could under the circumstances. At least on a temporary basis. By mid-afternoon I noticed that Karen had become very quiet and realized she was thinking about having to fly back to Houston tomorrow. Extremely hard on her. She is torn between the obligation of mother and wife. Once again, I told her to stay here in Michigan with the kids and reassured her that I would be alright. She won't hear of it. She says emphatically, "The kids will be okay until WE get home." Saying this aloud appears to help her believe its credibility. I love her and it torments me to helplessly watch this inner struggle she encounters so often. In my eyes, the sacrifice on Karen's part is greater than mine because I HAVE TO BE preoccupied with battling the cancerous tumor in my abdomen. My choice is justified. My choice is understandable. Karen's choice is not that simple or cut and dried. I'm too tired to think anymore tonight, much less write. Tomorrow is my final day at home so I want to be up early. Until then.

•DAY 40: SATURDAY, APRIL 15, 1989 — 7:00 A.M.
Good morning. The sun is out and it is the start of a beautiful day. Arose at 5:15 a.m. to take Ricky and one of his friends into

the printing plant to sort and bundle newspapers. This is a part-time job for our son and gives him spending money while it teaches responsibility. He is an excellent worker and picks up on learning new things quickly. Melissa, our oldest daughter, just went to take her A.C.T. tests. The A.C.T. is a college entrance requirement. She is nervous but am sure she will do fine. Melissa applies herself academically and is a good student. She'll be a senior next year. Doesn't seem possible. Feel like it was only a couple of years ago that I was changing diapers and hauling our kids around in car seats. Although I've kept my aches to myself since arriving home, the stomach cramps are severe this morning and my left leg is numb. The numbness disturbs me. Makes me speculate that the tumor is growing and pinching off the blood supply from the vena cava. Trying hard not to dwell on it and let Logo worry about this new problem when we get back to Houston. In four short hours we board for our return flight. Can hear the rest of the household stirring. Will record more entries later if time allows. One last thought: Very conscious of not wanting to leave home and return to Texas. My innate responsibleness is riddling me with guilt over "abandoning" the kids again. The feeling of guilt will fade but the pain of distant separation will not.

5:20 P.M. — We're back in Houston. Arrived at Hobby Airport about 3:00 p.m. Had a smooth flight, if there is such a thing. It was sunny and a splendid 72 degrees when we landed. The trip home to Michigan shed light on a lot of problems. Some present already, some to come. Karen and I confronted the REASON for the problems [my sickness] and trust that our approach diffused part of the tension. We reestablished some old rules and added some new guidelines at the old home-stead. Our decisions weren't entirely popular with the kids but they were necessary. Anyway, it was fantastic being home and the pleasing memories are still fresh in my mind. We arrived at our apartment around 4:00 p.m. After unpacking, the first chore on our agenda was to retrieve mail. In our absence we had accumulated quite a pile of letters. Karen said there were over 50 pieces of mail as she placed them all on our dining table. She was all teary-eyed as she said, "We are truly blessed with so much love represented here. It's S-O-O-O overwhelming. I hope we've earned it through the years because I feel so indebted to S-O-O-O many people. Thank God for our many, many blessings." This mail was our lifeline connection with home. It represented a support system we had not counted on but increasingly looked forward to each day.

9:00 P.M. — Just returned from a strenuous walk on the jogging path. Attempted a couple of times to jog very slowly. Karen Marie still opening and reading mail so have left her alone to enjoy the contents. Much pain tonight. My left leg is really aching and goes numb off and on. This appears to be a "new" but lasting side effect. Noticed it for the first time while back in Michigan. It definitely caught me unawares. Left arm is tingling like it's asleep as I write. Cramps got bad in late afternoon but have eased in the last hour and a half. As I walked tonight felt burdened by the fact that we're going to have extreme money problems in the near future. Trying not to worry about it but the truth is that I've always been the breadwinner and provider for my family. Awfully difficult to fulfill that responsibility from a hospital bed. This dilemma presents much self-imposed pressure. Karen wants to read me some of the loving, inspirational mail we received. Offers a happy note to end today's activities on. Supposed to be readmitted to M.D. Anderson tomorrow so it is time to focus on the battle once more. Think shrink and pleasant dreams.

•DAY 41: SUNDAY, APRIL 16, 1989 — 8:05 A.M.
Not difficult to tell we're back in Houston. Same dark thoughts of recent plagued my mind much of the night. Even the halcion sleeping tablets I took did not help. Abdomen pain woke me off and on as I fought tumor enlargement, spreading, reoccurrence, and terminal diagnosis in fitful dreams that lasted well past 3:00 a.m. Am waging quite a war against my unconscious mind. The recurring, ugly dreams seem to have the advantage at night and my positive speech and actions are superior during the day. Since I'm awake more than I'm asleep — I MUST be winning. In case you haven't noticed, a little humor is a mandatory requirement

for our daily health and welfare. Even poorly contrived humor. Humor adds spice and spice adds life. And LIFE is what I'm trying to maintain; mine to be specific.

10:10 P.M. — It's Sunday in Houston and we have been checked into M.D. Anderson since 12:30 p.m. Ended up in room 9015 which is Kevin "M's" old room. Not exactly the *Conrad Hilton* for accommodations, yet it has become our 2nd home. As we got into our room and settled, Karen and I both were aware of an intense gloom hanging over the 9th floor. Then we heard crying on the other side of the hall. Sid "P" had died at approximately 11:00 a.m. this morning and his family was still grieving for him. Sid lost a two-year battle with testicular non-seminoma cancer. He died directly from uncontrollable metastasizing. Very sad beginning to our debut back in the hospital. Logo and Dr. Ziegler looked worn out when they came by our room. I think Sid "P's" death was weighing heavy on both of them. He had been Logo's patient for quite some time. From my own observations, had concluded a while back that no matter how the doctors attempted to keep their professional distance, a certain bond and attachment did exist between patient and doctor. And some more than others. After all, they are both human beings before they are ever doctor and patient. Compassion is the key ingredient to these special few doctors who rise above the rest of their peers in patient empathy; it is also the Achilles heel which makes them emotionally vulnerable. In my estimation, Dr. Christopher J. Logothetis is one of those special doctors. Karen agrees with my estimation of Logo wholeheartedly. Kevin "M" was readmitted to our floor around 2:00 p.m. He introduced us to his sister, Brenda. She's also from the fine state of Texas and is going to stay with him through his 3rd chemo treatment. Kevin appeared rested and sounded good. Certainly looked better than he did when he left here 10 days ago. Another example of home environment doing wonders for recuperation. Getting late and we're beat. Until tomorrow.

MIDNIGHT — Can't sleep so went to the nursing station computer and ran my own lab count readout. My AFP was down to 32.8 and the rest of my counts looked stable. Undeniably good news. Oops, I'm playing doctor again! Reminds me, earlier today we ran into Larry "G" from Michigan. During our absence from the hospital his condition had apparently worsened because his sister was pushing him through the halls in a wheelchair. A newly discovered tumor in his femur bone had severely reduced his mobility. He stopped long enough to explain that his wife, Sissy [this is a family nickname for Bernadette], had to rush home to her father's funeral. Sissy's father was 82 years old. Felt sorry for Larry. His chalky complexion highlighted the panicked expression on his face. I'm sure he was kind of lost without his wife present to support and nurture him. Sissy is due back in two days. Overall, am glad to be on this floor because we know all the nurses and most of the patients but that familiarity can also be a drawback. The empathy sometimes leaves our own attitudes and emotions dangerously in harm's way. Sid "P" was under 30 years old with a new, young wife. His death seems so utterly unfair. Will be almost impossible to sleep with all these morbid thoughts running through my head. Depressing, to say the least. Need to concentrate on positive imaging and relax. Sleep is rest and I'm going to need all the rest I can grab for this next session of chemotherapy. Goodnight once again.

•*DAY 42: MONDAY, APRIL 17, 1989 — 7:45 A.M.*
Could possibly begin chemo treatment today. Depends on my blood counts. Feel decent and want to start as soon as possible. They just finished drawing my blood. Normally, the blood work is done between 5:30 and 6:30 a.m. See what happens? Leave for 3 days and everything goes to hell!
8:35 P.M. — We took a long, lazy walk this afternoon. Got quite a bit of sun as we warmed our attitudes and bodies. The telephone is not ringing much yet. Called home briefly yesterday and gave them our new room number and phone number. Kevin "M" started his chemo course at around 3:00 p.m. Logo came in at 5:15 p.m. and informed me that my counts were low in three areas. Thus, I would not begin treatment for another day at least. Am disappointed but honestly did not feel I would be able to start today. Cramps

are hitting me pretty hard right now. Don't think I'll ever get accustomed to this stomach pain. Wish I could grab onto something and just squeeze until the pain disappears. But that's what it is — a wish. Carl "M", a patient mentioned previously, ordered a pizza for us early this evening. The pizza had thin crust and tasted delicious. The sauce was extra spicy but still can only give it an "8" [on a scale of 1 to 10] versus our pizza in Michigan. Karen and I have been reading. I'm browsing a small religious handbook that our sister-in-law sent and Karen is deeply entrenched in one of her Harlequin romances. We're both extremely tired for some reason. Must be delayed jet lag, eh? We just looked up and said at the same time, "I miss the kids." That's what happens when you're married for so many years, you begin to think, talk and even look alike. We laughed and shared some fond memories of us and the kids. Time to get back to business. Need to start focusing on believing this tumor is going to shrink and believing I am NOT going to have any complications. On that note...we'll call it a day for my journal entries.

Chapter 8

THE REMAINING TREATMENTS

At this point, I am returning to the narrative form of writing. Primarily for two reasons. One: to avoid the repetitive circumstances and trivial details unavoidable with a journal format. Two: to accent the subtle changes in my attitude and perspective occurring weekly and even daily through the final three courses of chemo. My search for reassurances that neither doctors, medicine, nor myself could give were leading me to God and towards peace of mind. These next three courses of chemotherapy are the catalyst that started me on the way to comprehending that Rick Rockman Jr. did not have the final say on how this cancer fight would ultimately be decided. Frankly, this is when I began to discover, in my own words, that you *treat* cancer with medicine and *beat* cancer with God.

3rd SESSION: CISCA II AGAIN
APRIL 18, 1989 THRU MAY 11, 1989 — 23 DAYS

I began my 3rd course of chemo on April 18, 1989 at 6:30 p.m. Once again, went 23 days between treatments instead of the 21 day timetable. My low neutrophil count is what delayed starting the treatment on time. When I did begin the 3rd treatment my white blood cells [neutrophils] were still quite low. The white blood cell count is supposed to be at least 1500 and they were only registering 700. Medically, a level that reads 1500 for neutrophils indicates a relatively safe point at which chemo can be administered. Dr. Logothetis knew I was chomping at the bit to get started and I think he felt any more delay would hurt me more in the long run than it could help me in the short run. Logo took a chance. His roll of the dice ended up being sound judgement because I came through the session with no complications. Like most things in life, results are the final analysis on any judgement calls. My results were excellent. No viruses, no infections, no blood transfusions—no complications. The sum total equals a good judgement call on Logo's part.

Chemotherapy during this session consisted of a repeat of the Cisca II series. This entailed cytoxin, adriamycin and cisplatin being administered again over a 72-hour period. For this dose of cisplatin, my marathon vomiting session ONLY lasted five hours. The episode left me terribly drained and required over a week to regain any semblance of energy and strength. Through this course of chemo many of the same side effects plagued me as before. I was still besieged by the severe stomach cramps and constant muscle aches. Intermittently, I was dealing with headaches, earaches, fever and spells of extreme sweating. On top of these usual side effects was a new point of concern. My left leg and left arm were continuing to sporadically go numb and would throb with pain as I tried to shake feeling back into them. This hindered my walking at times and vastly disrupted my nighttime sleeping. Coping with this apparent vinblastine side effect became a daily chore. When I described the numbness and aching pain to Logo he did not seem surprised. With that reaction I decided that he had seen this side effect in other patients besides me and I might have to put up with it awhile. Little did I know how long "awhile" would end up being.

About this time is when I began reading two small handbooks our sister-in-law, Laura, had sent to us in the mail. They were written by a man named Kenneth E. Hagin, who is a non-denominational minister, born and raised in the state of Texas. These booklets fell into the Christian literature category. They were written for the express purpose of combatting the helplessness that all of us feel at one time or another during our everyday lives. Hagin would refer to scripture quotes from the Bible, then he would translate and explain. One of the first problems I encountered was that the author kept referring to "the Word." This captured my curiosity. If nothing else I wanted to discover what this so-called "word" was that Hagin repeatedly referred to in his booklet. About halfway through the booklet titled *God's Medicine* I figured out that "the Word" was nothing more than a synonym for the Bible. Hagin emphatically stated that the Bible IS the word of God. That's Bible as in the kind found in church, many homes and most hotels. It was so simple I couldn't believe that I'd never heard the term previously.

As I scanned the other small booklet one particular paragraph stuck in my mind. Kenneth E. Hagin maintained, "The Bible is a mystery book until we find the key that opens it. Then it ceases to be a mystery and becomes a message. There are two words which open up the Bible to our understanding — and those two words are LIFE and DEATH." These seemed like strong, sensible words and carried with them the credibility of a man who claimed to have been reading the Bible for over 50 years. Mr. Hagin's common sense explanations were easier to understand than the scriptural quotes he was using and translating. The statement on life and death grabbed my attention because that was what I was obviously engulfed in — a struggle for my life.

I was skeptical as I read some of the things Mr. Hagin stated with authority and conviction. He touched on everything from spiritual salvation to physical healing in a miniature 30 page handbook. Some I could not understand. Some I didn't want to believe. Some sounded like pure nonsense to my educated ears. The fact remained, as I read some of the biblical quotes he had selected I felt a temporary calm envelop my senses, a kind of peaceful strength. It was a fleeting sensation but I noticed it...so it must have been real. After a few more minutes of reading, I put the books down and went for a walk. At this point, the Bible and its contents were still a mystery to me. And if there indeed was a message, it remained unclear. Thinking had usually come easier and seemed clearer when I was alone in the sunshine or night air; so that's where I headed as I pondered some of Hagin's ideas.

With some of the well-meaning but far out literature we had recently been sent from an assortment of individuals, I'm surprised I even opened those Kenneth Hagin booklets. If Laura hadn't asked me about reading them during a phone conversation, I'm sure they would have ended up in a bag with many other well-meaning books we'd received. I'd already had bad experiences with some of the literature directed our way. Because of this, almost two weeks earlier I had adamantly informed Karen that I was not reading any more of the pamphlets or books sent to us. Many of them confused me with their so-called cancer cures. A few of them irritated me with their approach. Some of the concepts surrounding disease and sickness ascribed to by well-meaning individuals upset me to the point of disgust. A prime example is one book which was mailed to me by a friend. Its main point centered on the theme of accepting God's divine plan for mankind's redemption, health and welfare. The author, a Baptist minister, had some very peculiar ideas about the origin of sickness and disease. He was of the firm conviction that anyone stricken with cancer or another terminal disease should be able to say, "Thank you, God, for choosing me to be blessed with this glorious burden." I guess he figured that God designated those of us who are [or will be] afflicted with disease as His chosen few. Maybe this minister figured that sickness and disease were part of God's overall plan to humble mankind. Something along the lines of the chosen martyr theory, "Thanks God, for choosing me to suffer for your eternal glory."

Needless to say, I had a major problem with this kind of thinking. From day one, I had never blamed God for the tumor found in me. So, if I didn't blame God for my cancer, how in the world could I possibly thank God for the large, malignant tumor sitting in my abdomen. The answer I quickly arrived at was that I COULDN'T and SHOULDN'T. Reading episodes like this were similar to drinking diet pop; they left a definite after taste, one which I did not like at all. Hence, my attitude concerning material sent to us from friends and acquaintances evolved. It was much safer to read and stay busy with familiar, comfortable sources of inspiration. These little pamphlets by Kenneth Hagin seemed to be the exception. They offered positive hope and were presented in a down-home, earthy manner which I could understand. I was glad Laura had embarrassed me into reading the two Hagin booklets. They offered hope from an unexpected source and subtly directed me towards faith. Faith in the comfort of those words. His method of presenting these selected Bible quotes stimulated my curiosity and touched my common sense nerve endings. Hagin's handbooks made me ask myself soul-searching questions as I groped with the accuracy of his translations.

The God which I grew up praying to was an all-knowing, merciful and compassionate God. A God to be worshipped out of love, not fear. I needed and wanted God as an ally against this thing called cancer. With NO GUARANTEES being offered FROM ANY OTHER SOURCES it seemed natural to look skyward for help. Night after night, one of the last conscious thoughts I repeated to myself prior to sleep was that our God designed and desired for us to be healthy in body and spirit. I strived to believe this and said it to myself often throughout a day. Figuring once more, that if I repeated something enough times it would become established in my head and heart. To make a long story short, some of the literature sent to us was negative to my cause and the incorporated belief that God wanted all of us healthy. It was sent with good intentions but it was NOT for me. Literature like I mentioned earlier was detrimental to my whole outlook. Therefore, I avoided it like the plague whenever possible.

Back to the exception to my reading rule. The Kenneth Hagin booklets had impressed upon me two scriptures that I began to recite to myself and try to believe. The first one was *1 Peter 2:24* which ended with the words: "**... by whose stripes we were HEALED.**" Hagin insisted that this "healing" included disease and was a promise already fulfilled which was meant for every person on earth. The second biblical quote was *Mark 11:24:*

> **Whatever you ask in prayer, believe that you have received it and it will be yours.**

Powerful words and ones that I enjoyed hearing. But I cannot honestly say I even slightly believed them at first. For one, they sounded too good to be true. Whoever heard of getting what you ask for just because you believe it's rightfully yours? For another, doubts kept creeping into my mind suggesting that maybe this Hagin fella just interpreted the Bible to his own suiting. The scriptural quotes seemed to line up with positive thinking, that's the only reason I considered them as an aid at the time. It would do until I could find something better or grasp their meaning on my own. I continued to pick the booklets up and study them whenever I got the chance. Strangely, even though the words and their meaning didn't sink in immediately, whenever I finished reading them I continued to feel more at peace with myself. The fleeting inner peace also seemed to accent the fact that my battle was strictly personal. It involved me against cancer...and God as a possible ally. With this realization, it was definitely something to think about and consider.

On the second day of treatment, as I was taking adriamycin intravenously, a little excitement interrupted our day. I normally took morning walks. Sometimes with Karen Marie and sometimes without. This particular morning she did not accompany me. The previous night had been a restless one. I'd fought severe stomach cramps and muscle aches in my neck and shoulders much of the night. Besides the pain, I had to contend with the same old dark, ugly thoughts that usually haunted me when I couldn't sleep. On these nights, I just stared at the ceiling wide-eyed and wide awake. Consequently, restless nights would usually leave me quite tired in the morning.

Following this uneasy night, I took my usual morning walk around the concourse. After one lap I spotted a place on the lawn to sit down and rest. With the sun beating down on me and feeling good to my aching body I slowly laid back on the lawn. I'd parked my I.V. cart [complete with chemo drugs and pump] on the grass next to my head. Needing some quiet time, I pulled my baseball cap down over my eyes and gradually drifted off into never-never land. All of a sudden I groggily heard the beeper on my pump sounding and this computer voice saying, *"Help, air in line! Help, air in line!"* Startled, I tipped my cap back to find out what all the commotion was about. When I peered out I saw two ladies and a security guard staring at me. The first thing I heard over the beeping of my I.V. pump was the tallest lady telling the other lady, "See, I told you he wasn't dead."

The candid remark put a smile on my face. As I regained my sleepy senses and stood up I verbally confirmed for the ladies that they were correct, I wasn't dead. I had been sleeping sound and did not hear the I.V. pump alarm start beeping. The beeping sound and computer voice hollering for help had scared them to the point they went and harnessed a security guard to find out if I was alive or dead. They were visitors and apparently new to the M.D. Anderson facility. I chuckled and then thanked them for their concern. From there I got me and my I.V. cart back on the sidewalk and headed for the 9th floor nurses station. Figured if I kept moving, at least nobody would think I was dead again. My trek back to the 9th floor did not go unnoticed. About every 30 seconds the pump alarm would give another loud beep and the computer voice would holler "Help" one more time. Many self-conscious looks were coming my way as I scurried past people in the hallway and elevators. Me and my beeping pump seemed to make everyone nervous. This certainly didn't aid my efforts to keep a low profile until I could get the crazy thing back to my floor and fixed. When I eventually got back in my room and told Karen about the incident we shared a good belly laugh. The humor was good medicine for both of us and spiced up a rather routine day.

During my 3rd course of chemo I saw and kept track of many of the other patients whom I had befriended. Kevin "M" was developing into a real friend. Our sessions of scheduled chemotherapy continued to overlap so we were always within one or two days of starting or ending together. Even the prescribed chemo was the same at this point. When Kevin was taking a course of Cisca II, so was I. And when I was receiving a course of VB4, likewise for Kevin. We compared side effects, symptoms, progress and most importantly, speculated when we would be finished taking chemo. Our

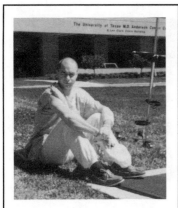

Taking a break during one of my walking sessions.

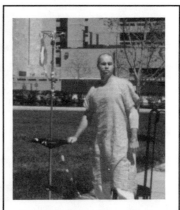

A partial view of my everyday walking route.

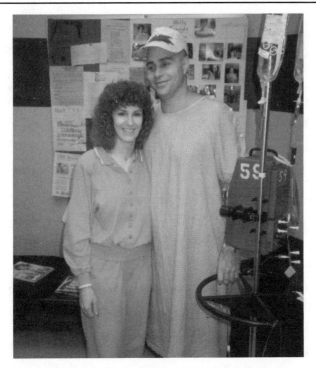

Karen and me posing for Kevin and Tina "M's" photo album.

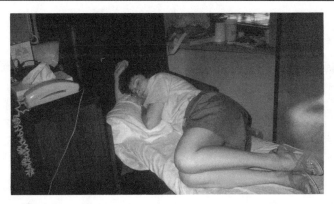

Karen napping. The fold-out chair served as her bed for six long months.

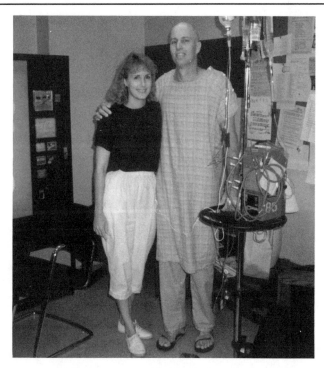

Kevin and Tina return the favor by posing for our snapshot.

similar diagnosis and plight allowed us to share some very sincere moments where we exchanged expectations, humor and even reservations whenever we got together.

Some of the other patients weren't nearly as fortunate as Kevin and myself. On Sunday, April 30th, Larry "G" had died. In our absence from the hospital Larry had been moved to I.C.U. and lost his battle to cancer while in the Intensive Care Unit. Karen and I stumbled onto this information when we tried to find what floor he had been moved to through a computer check. The news saddened us both. If you recall, Larry and his wife, Sissy, were from our home state of Michigan. Larry succumbed to renal cell carcinoma which had metastasized rapidly. We had come to know them quite well and our sincere sympathy went out to Larry's wife and children.

The same day we saw the wife of another patient and she informed us that her husband underwent emergency surgery for a bowel obstruction and was on a different floor than when we visited them last. Dwight and Elizabeth "P" have been mentioned previously. They are middle-aged with all their children grown and gone. Like Karen and me, they hailed from the Midwest part of the United States and called Indiana home. Their struggle with cancer had led them to Houston and M.D. Anderson just as ours had. They were extremely nice, friendly people and we hated to see them facing this latest complication. Dwight's chemo treatment was halted until he recuperated from the surgery. Once more, we realized how lucky I was in comparison.

A few days later we crossed paths with two other patients mentioned earlier. We bumped into Carl "M" in the Lutheran wing lobby as he was headed out the door to catch a bus. Carl was going home to Missouri. Blood tests indicated that cancer was still somewhere in his body but M.D. Anderson had done about all they medically could for him. Carl said he was headed home to take care of some personal matters and would worry about cancer later. After seeing Carl we headed up to the 9th floor nurses station to get some supplies for Karen to administer heparin locks. As stated previously, heparin is the solution used once a day to keep the medport line in my arm from clotting with blood. When not being infused with chemo the heparin is a daily task. While there, Vince "M's" room door was open so I stopped to chat with him as Karen visited with some of the nurses. Vince was fighting mouth sores and an infection that were compliments of his latest chemo course. Despite this, his spirits seemed good. Vince is an attorney from New Jersey. A month earlier, he had shared part of his cancer story with me. It could only be described as a horror story in misdiagnosis and misjudgment originating with treatment in his home state. Never heard him complain even though he had been fighting testicular non-seminoma cancer for well over a year. Vince and his wife, Gloria, had an apartment in the same complex we did. We both promised to try to get together if we were ever out of the hospital at the same time. Our conversation ended with that promise of future rendezvous.

As I related earlier, this course of chemotherapy left me extremely weak and tired. Following chemo infusion, Karen and I spent ten days in our apartment. This was actually the first extended period of time we had spent out of the hospital and at the apartment together. Prior to this, a few 4-hour passes had been the extent of our apartment living. By the end of this ten days I was beginning to get some strength and vitality back.

I came to the conclusion during this session that strength breeds boldness and confidence; while weakness breeds fear and frustration. It was a daily struggle to fend off the nagging physical weakness and remain mentally prepared to fight the symptoms of cancer and side effects of chemo. Slowly, I regained command of my body.

There was a paved jogging path near our apartment complex that was in easy walking distance and ran along Houston's Braes Bayou. The bayou was a small stream with concrete banks which meandered through the Southwest portion of outer Houston. Near dusk each night, We would take brisk walks along this well used path. Karen would get in her "shopping" stride and really stretch it out. A couple of times I even tried to jog. Gradually, I worked my way up to almost a mile of slow motion jogging. For the most part during these evening excursions, we would people watch and chit-chat as many other Houstonites biked, jogged and roller bladed past us on the asphalt route. The walks qualified as light exercise and were a refreshing change which got us out of the apartment for awhile. All too soon, our apartment stay was up and it was time to head back to M.D. Anderson for admission.

Being away from the hospital for those ten days, some of my strength and stamina had returned. I was just starting to feel human again, so we knew it was time to check back into the hospital for my next course of chemo. We had both become accustomed to the fact that my body never completely recovered from one chemo session before it was time to start another. With chemotherapy, this was just one more fact of...life in the cancer lane!

4th SESSION: VB IV AGAIN
MAY 12, 1989 THRU JUNE 2, 1989 — 21 DAYS

Prior to being admitted as an in-patient for the fourth course of chemotherapy I was put through another battery of tests. At this stage of treatment the tests were to compare tumor activity against past test results. I underwent another C.A.T. scan, spirometry test, gallium scan, full range blood work, chest and abdomen x-rays and finally, an ultra sound. This took two full days to accomplish. When we were eventually re-admitted it was only to find that my attending physician, Dr. Logothetis, was still on maternity leave. His wife had delivered a healthy baby boy on April 21st. This was their first born and they were proud, new parents. Logo was due back any day and that was fine with me since I couldn't start the next session without his O.K. and supervision.

On May 9, 1989, the day after we were officially admitted onto M.D. Anderson's 6th floor, Logo appeared for his normal rounds. He was still beaming over the birth of his newborn son. That morning he spent over an hour with us explaining my recent test results and answering questions.

This was part of the approach that made Dr. Logothetis special to Karen and me. Even when it seemed he was pressed for time, he TOOK THE TIME anyway.

Logo brought us up to date on the test results and laid out the tentative game plan. He was still very concerned about a primary site being confirmed. His concern was purely medical on this point. He did not want to treat me, send me home, and then get me back in a few months because an overlooked primary site was still emitting cancer cells. My concern was purely personal. I did not want ANY part of my body removed through surgery that did not absolutely have to be removed. That feeling certainly included my testicles. Especially, when there was so much speculation as to which one, if either, was the primary site. Logo put the issue to bed by saying we would worry about it later, after all chemo treatments were completed.

He did have some good news for us that morning. My AFP count, the blood marker that indicates cancer cells in the body, was down to 8.6. This was a huge decline from the 381.6 AFP count I had when I showed up at M.D. Anderson back in February '89. As I related previously, for my blood to be considered medically free of cancer the AFP count had to go below 5 and stay there. This number 5 represented an arbitrary figure which Logo and the rest of M.D. Anderson's physicians utilized. The number was purposely low. It demanded a smaller margin of error in the cancer victim's blood analysis. My AFP was headed there and that was great news.

During this informal discussion between Logo, Karen and me, the size of the tumor itself slipped out. Logo explained that at its largest point of penetration the dimensions had been 6-7 inches wide and almost 18 inches long. I was astonished! I had always known it was big but I had no idea that it was THAT big. Glad I didn't!

One more area of concern which Logo touched on that morning was the possibility that my vena cava and aorta were severely damaged. There were indications that the cancerous tumor had eroded the walls of both these large veins which run along the spine. Logo carefully stated that if this proved to be the case then during post-chemo surgery a medical team would have to rebuild the veins with a fine, synthetic mesh. The implication was clear to me...this would be a major complication if the scenario materialized. Logo's manner and the inflection of his voice while explaining confirmed my apprehension. This could be very serious.

The discussion ended with all of us understanding that I had to get through at least two more courses of chemo and then prepare for surgery. Logo casually hinted that the next two courses could be difficult. This information went in one ear and out the other at the time. But, within a week of that statement I would realize just how prophetic Logo's words of caution were.

At the very beginning of this 4th chemo session I received a book in the mail from one of my close friends back in Michigan. As teenagers, we had bought our first motorcycles together. Dan sent a short letter accompanying the book. He explained that he knew I wasn't reading a lot of the material sent to me because of its negative impact. But, he thought maybe I'd get something out of this one. The name of the book was *Healed of Cancer* and it was written by a minister's wife. Her name was Dodie Osteen. Five years before the book was published in 1986, she had been diagnosed with incurable liver cancer. Dodie Osteen claimed that by the healing grace of God she had beaten her imminent death sentence.

Out of curiosity and friendship, I picked the book up to browse through it and fulfill my obligation to Dan. I didn't put the book down again until I had finished reading it from cover to cover. From the first paragraph, it inspired me with the personal testimony that cancer can be beaten. It was full of personalized Bible quotes and Dodie's own agonizing story. Her down to earth message was crystal clear. She stated without a doubt that faith in God, and his word, were the only reason she was alive today. Dodie Osteen was [and is] a confirmed "miracle healing." Two different medical doctors went on record supporting her claim that she was cancer free everywhere in her body. They attested to the medical fact that at her stage of metastatic liver cancer [diagnosis and prognosis from December 1981] the most she could have hoped for, with the benefit of medicine, was 3-6 months to live. Today, she is an active, vibrant picture of health. [I can attest to that personally because I met and talked with her in July of 1989.]

The really amazing part of the Dodie Osteen story was that she and her husband, John, opted for NO treatment. Doctors had told her that even with chemotherapy they could not guarantee the prolonging of her life. The Osteens chose God as their doctor and went home from the hospital to fight cancer with God's medicine. They fought their battle armed only with the healing scriptures contained in the Bible and their faith in those words.

After reading Mrs. Osteen's book I was convinced that if she could beat cancer WITHOUT treatment and God's word, I could most certainly beat it WITH treatment and God's word. The only thing I forgot to take into consideration at this point was the fact that I did not quite have Dodie Osteen's degree of conquering faith. Actually, I wasn't even close to possessing her kind of unshakable trust in God. I wanted it and I was trying to get it, but it wasn't quite there yet. Not by any stretch of the imagination was it there yet. I was still holding on to the last remnants of the idea that I ALONE would beat cancer and get the assurances and guarantees my mind was demanding. Stubbornly, I just couldn't relinquish one more effort to control my own destiny. Could not fully accept the idea that my ultimate fate might be better off in someone else's hands. Even if that someone else was God!

Between Kenneth Hagin's booklets and Dodie Osteen's book, the material gave me a start in the right direction. For me, the right direction had to include solutions such as: no primary site being found; physical assurances against metastasizing and spreading; and emotional guarantees of no reoccurrence. For me, the right direction had to lead to genuine peace of mind. Without realizing it, I was still looking for this peace of mind through the manifestation of my own wishful thinking.

Although my faith wasn't operating on full throttle yet, I knew in my heart God had to be the answer. It seemed like God had quietly watched as I searched everywhere on earth for the answers to defeat this disease. He had patiently waited as I looked for the inner peace to confront the words, "Mr.

Rockman, you have cancer." Next, he quietly watched as I dealt with the physical pain of the huge tumor and the terminal forecast. God must have known that my search was leading me to eventually look skyward, towards *Him* for that inner peace. As I reflect back, it seems God knew where I was headed; *He* just didn't know when I would decide to get there.

At 11:00 a.m., on Friday, May 12, 1989 I began my fourth course of chemo. The course started with a bag of vinblastine. It would be vinblastine staggered with bleomycin for the next five straight days. Each drug would again be administered in 24 hour time increments. These were the drugs that attacked my system so severely during the first course of VB4 back in April. They promoted mouth sores, infection, earaches and severe muscle aches. As if to confirm my negative anticipation, the chemo hadn't been pumping into my veins for 30 minutes before an intense headache set in. These drugs literally hurt me from head to foot.

Two (2) words best describe this fourth course of chemotherapy...pain and sickness. The ever present cramps became worse with each day. Logo was fairly certain that the tumor had loops around my bowels and was constricting them as it reacted violently to the chemo drugs. He felt this accounted for the intense cramps all across my lower abdomen. With the constant pain, I was taking dilaudid in pill form and hydromorphone intravenously for some relief. The pain medication brought with it new side effects. They were constipation, irritability and depression. It was difficult to rationalize the trade-off. Apparently, I had traded taking the edge off my cramping pain for these assorted other side effects. Plus, the large doses of pain medication made me sluggish and drowsy.

To make matters worse, what started out looking like a leg rash was now a full-fledged yeast infection reaching from my groin area to halfway down my thighs. My inner thighs were covered with large, open sores from the infection. Even worse to me, was the fact that heat and sweating compounded the irritation. That meant no more outdoor walks while the sun was shining or the humidity was heavy. If you are familiar with the weather in Houston, Texas [even in May] then you understand I was sidelined until the infection cleared up.

Backtracking a little, another minor mishap took place during this time frame. On the second day of treatment, I was walking outside on the concourse at a swift pace and carelessly hit a raised crack in the sidewalks with my I.V. stand. The bleomycin bottle flew off the I.V. pole [just missing my head] and broke into pieces at the base of the I.V. stand's rollers. As usual, when I didn't know what else to do I headed for the nurses station on my floor. On the way, I alerted security to the broken glass and continued my trek to the 6th floor. The chemo bottle shattering on the sidewalk had caused a small cut on my foot. This put the nurses into a slight tizzy so they paged Logo and told him what happened. Thirty minutes later he was in my room checking me over from head to foot. Logo wanted to see how much of the bleomycin had got on my skin. When he was finished he told me it was a good thing it had not happened with vinblastine because that can severely burn the skin. I looked at Logo and with more than a little sarcasm in my voice stated, "It's okay to pump this stuff through my veins but not to get it on my skin? No wonder I think this stuff is really poison." This incident was my last outdoors walk before the yeast infection halted my outside activities. The way things were going maybe it was a good thing.

Each dawn seemed to bring with it a new side effect and more pain. I was enduring the pain during the day and praying for strength and relief at night. Literally, every muscle in my body ached. My left side, especially arm and leg, was going numb more often and staying numb longer. The tips of my fingers and toes tingled with the same numbness. I was steadily losing weight and had no appetite. Frequently, I would run high temps for hours, then I'd have chills. This was also the session where Karen noticed that my memory began to act up. I would say something, then repeat it later because I did not remember ever saying it. Earaches and sweating would hit me at night and disappear during the day. Last, but most certainly not least, were the mouth sores. These were ugly, canker-like sores which set into my mouth and tongue on the ninth day of treatment. Admittedly, I was a big baby where these were concerned. Maybe because I had tried so hard to head them off. I had gargled and coated my mouth with Milk of Magnesia numerous times throughout each day. Now it seemed for naught. The fact remains that they were a painful frustration that I did not handle very well.

Without being melodramatic, the VB4 course of chemotherapy was extremely tough on me with its caustic drugs. Both mentally and physically. To add insult to injury, I recalled Logo's cautious warning concerning the next treatments. His subtle forewarning had literally gone in one ear and out the other. There was little comfort knowing I had been warned. At this phase, I was just trying to cope. To combat fatigue, depression and pain I utilized what had worked in the past. I kept as busy as possible with reading and walking. Much of my walking was inside the hospital for this session. Outdoor walks were my real choice but the yeast infection kept me penned up indoors. Since I couldn't walk outdoors, I did the next best thing and used my mind to take me places. Through mental imagery exercises, I visualized myself in healthy, everyday situations while besieging my mind with the same positive thoughts. And I never stopped privately praying. When you want something it's surprising how often you remember to call on God.

Near the end of this treatment I gave Karen a shock and myself a misapplied morale boost. It was late in the evening, and we were winding down another long, frustrating day. Between the mouth sores and cramps I was totally miserable. My limited ability to walk and exercise because of the infection had contributed greatly to the frustration. On this particular night, I felt compelled to tell Karen one of my innermost recurring thoughts. Out of nowhere I informed Karen, "It would be a lot easier to just roll over and lay here waiting to die." Her eyes got big as saucers and then she carefully said, "I've never thought of you as a quitter." I told her that I didn't mean I was giving up but that the statement was every bit accurate. She calmly replied, "Maybe it is but I don't enjoy hearing you talk that way." That was all it took to get me back on track and stop feeling sorry for myself.

By the completion of the fourth session my body was just plain beat up and my mind was totally exhausted. My eyes kind of told the tale. Karen described them as dull and uncharacteristically void. Chemo had zapped their customary sparkle. My weight was down to 159 pounds and I had been on hyperalimentation for eight days. Appetite was a non-existent urge. My skin color was pallid and gray toned. The yeast infection was about gone but the other many side effects were still wrestling with my body. The cramps and mouth sores continued to present the most pain and frustration. Despite all this I was actually doing better than some of my friends who were being treated. When I considered the pain and trauma these friends were facing it always seemed to put my problems back in perspective.

Besides the numerous events taking place at M.D. Anderson during my daily battle, much had been happening elsewhere in our lives. Back home, our two oldest girls were scheduled to go to the 1989 Fenton High School prom. I knew that missing this special event was quietly gnawing at Karen's mind so I suggested she fly home for a few days around prom time. At first she balked but I convinced her that with two birthdays in May and the prom taking place, it would be time well-spent for her and the kids. Karen was hesitant to leave me alone and not completely comfortable with the timing when she considered the proposed trip.

Her decision received an assist when she discovered that my oldest sister and youngest brother planned to visit with me for a few days during the time frame she would be home. With this knowledge, she finally consented. We had decided to send her home on May 16th and have her return on May 24th. These dates would allow Karen and the kids to celebrate Melissa and Ricky's birthdays and accommodate the prom on May 20th. Under this schedule she'd be here with me to start my fourth session and return before it was completed. I'd miss her terribly but felt strongly that she should be home for some of the upcoming special events. Karen felt just as strongly that eight days was too long to be away from me. She was worried. Common sense was the deciding factor. Our kids needed one of us and I had no choice in the matter. We had agreed in the beginning that unless it was an absolute emergency the chemo sessions would not be delayed or interrupted. Thus, I stayed, Karen went.

On the 19th of May, my brother and sister arrived. Both came in about noon. Ron flew in from California and Deb arrived from Michigan. Karen had been home to Michigan for three days. Nightly, she was keeping me posted by phone. From the sounds of it she had her hands full dealing with our kids and their many activities. Her busy schedule at home was running into 18 hour days. From the sounds of her voice the hectic pace she was keeping was taking its toll. Karen didn't need to know that I had been sick and getting sicker since the day she left. After encouraging her to make the trip home I sure didn't want to drop any unneeded guilt on her head. There wasn't a single thing she could do to help. Events were going to run their course with or without her presence.

Actually, from the minute my 4th course started it had been a rough road to travel. Unfortunate timing for Ron and Deb's visit but they certainly didn't know how sick I was going to be during the treatment. Neither did I!

We secured a four hour pass so I could show Ron and Deb where the apartment was located. We even managed to take in a show in our short time away from the hospital. As it turned out it was good we got away from the hospital for those few hours. After our pass, the better portion of their three day visit was spent in my private room talking, reminiscing and watching me progress from sick to sicker. Ron and Deb looked healthy and well. In fact, they looked as healthy as I did sick. Most important to both of them was my current condition and welfare. I put their minds at ease as much as possible and tried not to let them know just how sick I felt during this treatment. I can still recall the look on their faces as the hospital went about its regular business and patients flowed in, out and past my room. Ron, bless his heart, was kind of shell-shocked. The sick faces, bald heads and the normal aura of oppression that goes with a hospital environment were contributing to his numbed look. Deb, trying to be a big sister, was taking all of the activity in and yet, not letting the oppressive atmosphere show on her. I was glad for their company and tried to be decent company myself. Looking back, I'm not sure I did very well.

Meanwhile, two of my patient friends had been admitted about the same time as me. They were both on the 9th floor of the Lutheran Building while I was on the 6th. Kevin "M" was in the hospital for the exact same course of chemo as myself. It was also his fourth treatment. He looked rested and his skin color appeared much better than the last time we had seen him. Eddie "T" was back in the hospital for his last course of chemo. This would be his fifth treatment. Eddie seldom discussed his prognosis other than to confirm that he had the same type of cancer I had. He was one of the few people I encountered who did not want to talk about their cancer. I never pushed this point. Cancer is a very personal battle and I always tried to be sensitive to everyone else's method of coping. Amazingly, Eddie still had not lost his hair. I told him he'd obviously never have to worry about being bald. Eddie and I came to the conclusion that if chemotherapy couldn't scalp him—even heredity didn't have a chance of stealing his hair.

Something very eerie occurred with Kevin on the day we began our fourth course of chemo treatment. I remember the exact scene like it was yesterday.

He came down to my floor before lunch and caught me alone in my room reading. One of our topics of conversation that late morning concerned the Intensive Care Unit. Both of us had noticed that when patients were sick enough to end up there they usually didn't come back. At least it was true of everyone we knew who had gone to I.C.U. All had died. We jokingly agreed that if either one of us ended up there it was time for our family to be notified and make a final visit. We small talked for a couple more minutes before Kevin announced he'd better return to his room in case his chemo was ready. Kevin had a different doctor than I did so his treatment was starting early in the afternoon while mine was scheduled for later that evening. As he was leaving my room Kevin stopped in the doorway, looked back, and said very seriously, "I have a bad feeling about this treatment, Rick. I don't know if I can get through it."

I replied, "C'mon Kevin, you'll make it easy. Especially when we're this close to finishing." He just looked at me, gave me a half-hearted smile and disappeared through the doorway. As soon as Kevin was out of sight our last exchange was out of my mind. At the time, I had no idea how foreboding Kevin's intuition would end up being. If I had, I like to think I would have handled our brief exchange much differently. Don't know if it would have changed the outcome but the effort could not have done any harm. Sometimes, guilt has tried to set in concerning this short conversation we had, but then I reconcile the circumstances in my mind by realizing that hindsight is always 20/20 vision.

True to his own premonition, by the next afternoon Kevin was already becoming very, very sick. Unsuspecting, I went up to his floor to see him in the early afternoon. When I came through the door and into his room I just stood there and gaped. The sight which greeted me was scary. Kevin, with five or six bags of medication, antibiotics and chemo hanging from his I.V. cart, was lying on his bed staring at the ceiling. Ringing his face were beads of sweat that clung to his forehead, cheeks and chin. He raised his hand and painfully pointed to his mouth as he slowly shook his head sideways. I knew he was telling me that his tongue and throat were full of sores and swollen to the point he could barely speak. Grotesquely, his feet and hands were beginning to turn black and blue and swell. This was an apparent chemo side effect I'd never witnessed or heard about. I couldn't believe this was the same person I had visited with 24 hours earlier. Standing there dumbfounded, I asked, "Kevin, what happened?" He looked at me with blank, staring eyes and slowly mumbled four words, "I told you so."

By this time, Kevin was not the only one having problems. Phil "C" had just come back in for treatment. He was a new friend. We'd met a few weeks before. His wife, Marjorie Ann, had hit it off well with Karen. The girls shared a common interest; getting their husbands cured and back home. Their friendship formed a bond that only the spouses of cancer patients would comprehend. It was a bond based on emotional commitment. A commitment to their spouse which I'd enjoyed through Karen since the very first day of this cancer nightmare. A commitment based on unconditional love and devotion. I was the beneficiary of that commitment from my wife and I sensed that Marjorie Ann gave Phil the same commitment. Karen and Marjorie Ann were typical of the many wives I encountered in the confines of M.D. Anderson. They stuck by their husbands for better or for worse...and that included confronting cancer.

On many occasions, I would look over at Karen as she kept vigil and see the pain and stress of my misfortune etched into her face. She was never granted the luxury of exposing her sometimes frayed emotions. Because she was the healthy one in our situation, she wasn't expected to be human. Her fears and weaknesses weren't allowed to come to the surface. She was expected to retain her composure and not bend to the stress AT ALL TIMES. Due to the emotional demands and commitment, I still believe that cancer is harder, in many aspects, on the spouse than it is on the cancer patient. On a daily basis, I tried to always keep in mind that Karen was suffering too. This perception often prevented me from feeling sorry for myself. That in itself was a blessing because I recognized from the very beginning that self-pity is a self-destructive, dead end street. Sometimes literally.

Phil's return was unexpected. He'd went home to Florida weeks earlier to regain his strength and gradually assume his normal duties. At that time, Phil's bladder cancer was supposedly in remission. His regular check-up is what revealed the latest cancer site. Now he was back at M.D. Anderson with another tumor[s] and different location. Apparently, the primary bladder site had metastasized. This time the malignancy was in his lung. Instead of having his check-up and returning home, he would be admitted again as a patient. Prior to this latest development, Phil had undergone intensive chemotherapy for months and finished up with 14 hours of surgery. In conjunction with the latest development he was informed right up front that the recent biopsy indicated this type of tumor to be resistant to chemotherapy. The only protocol M.D. Anderson could extend was experimental drugs. This new twist was a real downer. Phil had gone home under the hopeful impression his cancer fight was in the past and now he was once more fighting for his life in the present. I had always suspected that life was not fair. Phil's lousy predicament is what confirmed for me that *life is neither fair nor easy!*

Unconsciously, the medical status of my friends affected my personal outlook. We were an unrecognized fraternity. Simply put, if I did well through a treatment then other patients who knew me expected to do well. If I received positive test results, they expected good news from theirs. We were fighting separate battles but we were fighting the same enemy — cancer. Unintentionally, we fed off each other. This theory seemed to work in reverse just as vigorously. And at this point in time, the measuring stick was mired on the negative side. Eddie was depressed and would hardly speak. Kevin was so sick he could barely speak. Phil was trying to face the anguish of metastasizing and all its terminal implications. Suffice to say, their present condition did not help my overall outlook.

My outlook soon got a much needed face-lift. I received a beautiful surprise on May 31st around 9:00 p.m. My brother Craig flew into Houston unbeknownst to me. He set me up good. The phone rang in our room a little before 9:00 p.m. Texas time; it was Craig. We small talked for a few short minutes and then he said, "Hang on Rick, we must have a bad connection...I'm going to the phone in the kitchen." As I was [im]patiently waiting on the phone the door to my room flew open and in popped Craig with a grin ear-to-ear. He had called from the lobby of M.D. Anderson. My spirits had been low so Craig's unexpected appearance represented great timing and bouyed our spirits. The attitudes of both Karen and myself got an immediate overhaul. He looked absolutely great and said he had completed his radiation treatments. He was scheduled for a routine check up in July or August. This was fantastic news in itself.

We laughed and carried on for awhile before Karen reminded us it was getting late. She escorted Craig over to our apartment and got him settled in with the promise he could come back up to the hospital early in the morning.

The next day, Craig's surprise visit prompted a pass from Logo to leave the hospital for a few hours. Naturally, Karen wanted to shop and I, just as naturally, wanted to talk privately with my brother. We compromised with a trip to the huge Galleria mall located on the outskirts of Houston. While Karen shopped, Craig and I discussed family, business and old times. We did NOT talk about cancer. Besides, Logo would be in the following day and we would hear enough concerning cancer when he brought us up to date on my prognosis and upcoming surgery.

Time flew during Craig's visit. He was quite impressed with the M.D. Anderson facility and staff. On his second day in town, he finally got to meet Dr. Logothetis and Dr. Cox. If you recall, Dr. James Cox had played an important part in evaluating Craig's own cancer back in January of 1989. This visit gave Craig an opportunity to personally thank Dr. Cox for his involvement. Like me, he enjoyed the reassurance of putting a face and personality with the voice he had communicated with over the phone.

The trip for Craig had been made on a spur of the moment impulse. Three short days was all he could take off work. So, before we knew it, the time was up and Craig was headed back to Michigan. We enjoyed his company immensely. His presence had brought with it a revitalizing hint of home.

As close as we were, our personal battles with cancer had brought my brother and I even closer. Craig and his wife, Beth, remained in our thoughts and prayers every single day. I repeat, Karen and I NEVER forgot that he was fighting cancer also. Often, his cancer ordeal was overshadowed by the severity of mine. This seemed especially true because of the fact that I took treatment in Texas and he remained in Michigan. Texas was where I HAD TO BE because M.D. Anderson was one of the few institutions which had treated my rare form of cancer with any degree of success. People back home didn't seem to understand that Michigan was where Craig COULD BE because treatment was basically the same at all institutions for his type of cancer.

Remaining at home certainly didn't nullify or neutralize the impact of cancer on Craig's life. It just made mine seem worse. Craig's situation always reminded me that in this respect cancer is cancer. There is no good kind. It all kills. Some types are just more treatable than others.

On Friday, June 2, 1989 my fourth treatment was officially over. Although some of the severe side effects were still lingering on, my blood counts had remained surprisingly high. I looked and felt like death warmed over but the doctors go by blood tests for their evaluation, not looks and feelings. Good thing! Mentally, I was drained. Emotionally, I was exhausted. The only redeeming factor was that I was on schedule for going home. For all intents and purposes it appeared I would begin my next treatment on time. Hopefully, this would be the final dose of cisplatin to endure.

5th SESSION: CISCA II
JUNE 3, 1989 THRU JUNE 23, 1989 — 21 DAYS

Let's begin this session with a brief patient update. I didn't forget these people then so I certainly don't want you to now. By the beginning of June, our friend Phil "C" was taking chemotherapy again. His attitude was upbeat and his body had recovered enough to tolerate some more courses. Additional surgery was planned for him in 2-3 months. He was doing as well as he could under the trying circumstances. Karen and I felt nothing but sincere empathy for Phil and his wife.

My reclusive friend, Eddie "T", went home at the end of May. The day Eddie left he looked absolutely terrible. As he gathered his belongings from the hospital room his last remark to me was, "I JUST want to get out of here and go home." Believe me, I could definitely relate to that. The old cliche, "Home is where the heart is" had taken on new meaning for me months ago. Better than anyone I understood that Eddie wanted to recover from his last dose of chemo in the confines of his own friendly, familiar surroundings; otherwise known as home.

Poor Kevin. He ended up in I.C.U. and had an emergency

tracheotomy done. With the aid of the tracheotomy, Kevin was put on a respirator to help him breathe. This procedure probably saved his life. I say this because pneumonia seems to claim more victims than the cancer itself after a body is severely weakened by chemo. The respirator helped exercise Kevin's lungs and prevent pneumonia from getting a death grip. While in I.C.U. the swelling in his extremities got so bad that the skin on his feet and hands burst. Sounds unbelievable but it is "Oh, so true." Theoretically, Kevin had a radical reaction to the vinblastine and bleomycin chemo drugs which in turn attacked his nerve endings and muscle tissue. His fingers, toes, palms of the hands and soles of the feet sustained most of the damage. The doctors said if he recovered that he would have to undergo physical therapy. They offered no guarantees for a complete recovery, especially where Kevin's feet were concerned.

For almost three weeks of constant vigil, Kevin's wife, Tina, and immediate family shared shifts at the hospital around the clock. It was touch and go for quite a few days. Kevin was literally at death's door throughout those days. He's still very sick but with each new sunrise it looks as if he might be the first patient to survive a trip to Intensive Care. The first one that either of us are aware of, that is.

Our conversation about patients not making it back from I.C.U. has plagued me often during Kevin's stay there. Silently, I hoped that Kevin was too out of it to recall our negative appraisal. Bedridden, in his Intensive Care surroundings, remembering the conversation we had could only have made his situation worse.

Karen and I felt terribly helpless while Kevin was so dreadfully sick. Part of the helplessness stemmed from our close relationship with Kevin and his immediate family. Makes it harder to endure when you know someone personally. Knowing that he's a fighter had not eased our concern.

Kevin required more than toughness to get through these last few weeks. Seems like a fleet of guardian angels have been watching over him for much of his extended stay in I.C.U. It was truly a living nightmare for Kevin. All we could do at this stage was pray for his recovery and offer words of encouragement to his family. Against hospital regulations I did manage to sneak into the Intensive Care Unit, once with Karen and once alone. Kevin was only semi-conscious but thank God I could see he was alive. Karen has maintained for quite a few years that I'm not happy unless I'm violating some rule or guideline. Maybe she's right but in this instance the thrill was in seeing Kevin, not the rule breaking.

At 11:00 p.m. on Saturday, June 3rd I started my fifth treatment. Cisca II infused one more time. I had mixed emotions as I began this last course. As usual, I wanted to start so I could finish, but I knew my body was still dragging from the awful effects of the fourth treatment. Frankly, I wasn't sure I could take another course as severe as the previous one. So, for the last 3-4 days I had been preparing mentally for this session. I concentrated on prayers, positive imaging and going home. More PAR in other words. Logo had said that after chemo and before surgery I could go home for 4-5 weeks to allow my body to recover. I was pointing towards that time frame.

Cisca II is the treatment that takes a little over three days to administer. It's also the treatment that finishes up with nasty ol' cisplatin. Once again, cisplatin lived up to its morbid reputation of making one deathly sick. Although it was another bad episode of throwing up, in truth, it was much less severe than the previous two episodes. I ONLY vomited my insides out for 4 and a half hours this time. Plus, I seemed to recover faster after this session. Following the vomiting, I rested for about eight hours and then forced myself to get out of bed, go outside and walk. The recovery was probably speedier because I was focused on finishing the session and getting Karen and me on a plane headed back to Michigan. MY schedule said it was time to go home and be with our kids. Time to take a break from the grief of chemotherapy and hospitals. This was a timetable I was looking forward to meeting.

Medically, my prognosis was holding the line. Only a couple areas of anxiety were changed from the fourth course of chemo. For one thing, concern over a primary site [suspected source of the original tumor] had not been discussed in weeks. And that discussion had occurred at the conclusion of my 3rd treatment. Secondly, my AFP count was down to 4.8. My blood markers were conclusively considered normal. At last, no trace of cancer was evident in my bloodstream. It was officially under the norm of 5 which had been a mandatory requirement of Logo. All that remained was to take this session of chemo and continue to keep the AFP below that magic number of 5. How long? Forever, I hoped.

Finally, much to Logo's surprise, the tumor in my abdomen had shrunk some more. In past conversations, Logo had stated that he didn't think the tumor would shrink anymore. Despite these "don't get your hopes up too high" predictions, I'd always pray and use positive imaging to support my "shrinking" efforts.

Some of my mental imagery concerning tumor shrinkage was quite creative. I perfected the technique to the point where I could turn everyday activities into tumor shrinking exercises. For instance: On my daily walks I devised a "spool of yarn" visualization. This is where I'd mentally see the tumor as a large, black spool of yarn. As I walked the spool would unravel. The longer I walked, the smaller the spool [tumor] got. In my mind, the smaller the tumor, the deader and better. Within this scenario I'd unravelled many spools of yarn and dissolved my huge tumor many atime over the past weeks. The results surprised Logo and pleased us both.

The punishing mouth sores had finally disappeared. Cramps remained. Headaches, earaches and muscle aches had let up gradually. For the most part though, they too were gone. I continued to have the numbness and aching fingers to deal with. My hands and fingers were getting bad enough that I couldn't seem to write. This curbed my letter writing and journal notes. I dealt with it the best I could. Due to the numbness, I couldn't even read some of my entries in the journal. Now that's bad when you cannot read your own writing.

I hadn't neglected the prayer pattern I referred to in my third course of chemo. It was included in my personal PAR [Positive Action Routine] everyday. Even with the terribly rough time I had during the fourth course my pursuit of inner peace was a daily endeavor. The potential of God as this source was not forgotten. Quietly, to myself, I'd often repeated the healing words of scripture that Mr. Hagin and Mrs. Osteen had volunteered in their literature. These meditations always seemed to calm me down and take the edge off things. Many of my friends were the benefactors of my quiet time prayer pattern. Through the fourth session I had expended as many prayers on these individuals as I had on myself. This didn't necessarily qualify me for sainthood, but it did accent that when you can care about someone else's welfare yours will become much less intimidating. In the mental realm anyway, if not the physical.

Another surprise visitor appeared in Houston as we officially began the last course of chemotherapy. My mom arrived at 11:00 p.m. on Saturday, June 3, 1989. Unfortunately, she had experienced a delayed, turbulent flight into Houston and was mildly upset by the time she got to the hospital and up to our room. After talking for a few minutes she settled down and began to relax. She and my dad had been catapulted into the role of active parents again because we were stuck here, in Houston. Supervising our kids and house sitting was far more important to us than anything else they could volunteer. For this trip, my dad had remained at home to help keep an eye on the kids and tend to daily business.

The shock of seeing her oldest son 35 pounds lighter, bald-headed and sickly pale, eventually faded from mom's face as we talked. She had not seen me since the middle of February, back in Michigan. Our last visual contact had been the day prior to Karen and me leaving for Houston and the M.D. Anderson Clinic. At that time, I had been diagnosed with terminal cancer but had actually looked healthy and normal. Reflecting back to that moment makes me think of the old cliche, "Looks can be deceiving." It seemed like mom had prepared herself well for my P.O.W. [Prisoner of War] appearance before she arrived. After almost four months of separation it was terrific to see her.

The tanned, athletic look she had nurtured while wintering in Florida for several weeks made her look healthy and trim. Notwithstanding the fact that her two oldest sons were battling cancer, her attitude was upbeat. Mom was trying to be as strong emotionally as she appeared physically. Briefly, she brought us up to date on how and what everyone back home was doing. Soon after this update Karen sensed that the plane ride had worn mom out. She interrupted the conversation and reminded us all that we could discuss things more alertly in the morning. Karen offered to get the car and escort mom to our apartment before she collapsed from fatigue. We shipped her off to our apartment sometime after midnight. With five months of Texas driving under her belt, Karen was as familiar with much of Houston's locale as some of the taxicab drivers. Nevertheless, I always worried when she had to travel alone in Houston. Especially at night.

My mom's unannounced visit gave Karen a break from baby-sitting me every minute. She needed it. Although her crying spells had become less frequent, the separation from our children was wearing on her more and more. Mom's visit provided the opportunity to escape the depressing hospital routine for a few hours. They were able to work in a shopping trip one day and attend a cancer survivors' reunion picnic the following day. Karen even bought a couple of summer outfits during their shopping expedition instead of her usual window shopping. She and mom genuinely enjoyed the survivors' picnic. Karen would have liked for me to see and visit with some of these cancer survivors. She felt it would ease my mind since I had asked her quite a few times in the past, "Where are the people that beat cancer? How come I never talk or bump into any of the good story people?"

Before mom left for home she met Logo. This gave her the chance to question him at length on my prognosis and upcoming surgery. Logo's answers seemed to put her mind at ease and satisfy her motherly concerns. Mom headed back home on June 8th equipped with short-term answers and full of hope. Karen and I planned to be shortly behind her for OUR trip home.

Worth mentioning at this point is an incident that occurred in the cafeteria of M.D. Anderson. The day after I had finished receiving the final dose of Cisca II, I went out for my usual morning stroll. The cisplatin hangover effects had left me very weak but I managed to complete four rapid laps around the concourse sidewalk. Tired, I started back to the sixth floor. On the way back I decided to stop in the main floor cafeteria. Even though I couldn't eat the hospital food [or should I say wouldn't eat?], Karen needed some food and nourishment. Figured I'd tell her the evening menu and let her decide from there. Thanks to chemotherapy heightening my sense of smell the odors in the cafeteria usually made me instantly nauseated. Knowing this, I stood back as far as possible from the steaming food and tried to read the counter menu.

As I was looking over the menu a rather tall, middle-aged lady came into my line of vision. She continued to walk towards me as I read. With the lady still moving at me, I tried to peer around her body and see the menu. Before I realized it, she was standing directly in front of me, about two feet away from my face and staring into my eyes. After an awkward few seconds she matter-of-factly stated in a hoarse, low-pitched voice, "So, you've got the BIG 'C', huh."

I about fell over. It wasn't really a question, rather, it was more like an accusation. Not recognizing her face, all I could think of at that instant was, "What a stupid thing to say to me with a cafeteria full of so-called BIG 'C' patients."

Hoping this was an innocent mistake I glanced behind me to make sure she wasn't speaking to someone else. No one was within ten feet of us so I was out of luck there. The second thing I did was to self-consciously look all around me and see if anyone else had heard this nut. Everyone seemed to be going about their business.

I couldn't believe my luck! With one comment this mystery lady had me embarrassed and tongue-tied, all at once. Karen will attest to the fact that rarely am I at a loss for words. Well, I was here. Finally, I asked, "Lady, are you talking to me?"

Shaking her head up and down, she said in that same accusing tone, "Yes, honey, I *am* talking to you."

Now I was becoming defensive as I told her in no uncertain terms, "I don't even know you!...Yeah, I have cancer...The

BIG 'C' as you call it...what about it?"

This time she shook her head sideways and kind of smiled. For what seemed like an eternity, she just kept shaking her head and smiling. All I could do was stand there and stare back. Then, without another word, she turned around and slowly walked to the double door exit at the rear of the cafeteria. Every few steps she would look back at me over her shoulder and give that same smile. It was kind of a smirking sneer which implied she knew something that I evidently didn't.

After she vanished through the doorway I scanned the cafeteria once more and then began to smile. I just kept shaking my head and smiling as I looked around at the other cancer patients who were in the cafeteria at the time. All the while I kept thinking to myself, "Why me? There has to be 60-70 other patients right here with me. We all basically appear the same. We're bald-headed, hooked to an I.V. cart and downright skinny. Doesn't she know that EVERY patient in this hospital has the BIG 'C'? Who was that nut?"

When I returned to our room and shared the incident with Karen she was aghast. Suspiciously she asked me, "Are you sure you didn't know her from somewhere?" I told her that I was positive. No way would I have forgotten meeting this woman. Not knowing what to make of the circumstances all we could do was try to laugh it off and record it as one more bizarre event associated with my cancer fight. To this day, I do not have the slightest idea who that lady was or why she singled me out of the crowd to share her keen observation on cancer. I do know that she was weird and the circumstances were weird. I'm not sure I care to know anymore than that.

On the morning of June 10, 1989 Karen and I were finally flying back home for a month of recuperation time. The day before, Logo and his assistant, Betsy, had spent a long time lecturing us [more to the point ME] on the *can do's* and *cannot do's* to be followed while away from the hospital. They were supposed to be words of caution but the warning was unmistakable. I was reminded that my blood counts were low and would remain that way for at least another week to ten days. This fact meant that I was very susceptible to infections and any kind of cut or scratch could be dangerous. Another area of concern was where to go for treatment if I did have problems arise. Logo settled on an old Med school classmate who was practicing in Dearborn, Michigan. I agreed to check into the Dearborn connection once a week to have my blood monitored. Quite naturally, I also agreed to take it easy and nodded my head "yes" to all areas of concern. Knowing as I did so that the minute I felt the least bit human again I would probably do as I pleased.

Logo is a smart man and caring doctor, while I'm just a know-it-all set in his practiced ways. I think Logo suspected this as he tried to scare me into behaving. He must have realized my "I can handle it" attitude might get me into some serious trouble. Meaning unneeded complications. The fact of the matter is that I most likely would have agreed to any restrictions because all I wanted to do was get home. Our children, family and friends were waiting. Home and everything it stood for was waiting. Good-bye chemotherapy and hello Fenton, Michigan were utmost on my mind!

Chapter 9

SURGERY and RECOVERY

We landed at Detroit City Airport late in the afternoon. I can't describe how absolutely great it felt to be back in Michigan. My brother, Craig, picked us up at the Northwest Airlines terminal. Karen and I thanked God Almighty that we were home and would be able to spend some much needed time with our children. With anticipation, we looked forward to the 4-5 weeks of recovery time at home. Our hopes and expectations were high as Craig chauffeured us into the growing little city of Fenton. The only matter that tainted our drive home was my weakened state. Some of the same side effects were resolutely hanging on. Most notable were the stomach cramps and aching numbness in my left side limbs. The pain and discomfort prevented my elation at being home from always shining through. Everybody seemed to understand I wasn't 100 percent except me. As usual, I was my own worst critic.

My appetite was coming back, my hair wasn't. Karen had been noticing of late that my memory was becoming even worse. It appeared to be my short-term memory which was affected the most. She didn't say much when it happened but I would get quizzical stares from her sometimes as we talked which indicated the topic must have already been discussed. I just couldn't remember. The earaches which I'd tolerated for the last couple of months had given way to a steady ringing in my ears. I was starting to notice difficulty in separating sounds. If a conversation was taking place and there was any background noise at all the voices seemed to blend together. The result was that I could not tell who was saying what.

Lastly, my skin was showing small black and blue marks in quite a few places on my arms, legs and feet. The marks resembled bruises but were not caused by any kind of pressure to my skin. Compliments of chemotherapy, they just seemed to appear. For how long I didn't know.

Our homecoming was a jubilant affair. The first three or four days were spent renewing our parenthood with the kids. Some of the renewal went smooth and some went not-so-smooth. Karen and I both realized we had to reestablish our positions of authority and leadership. We hoped the kids realized as readily that love was the motivating force behind our efforts. Amidst this priority we visited with family and friends who were coming by the house in droves to show their sincere care and concern. With all the love and prayers coming our way, we never complained about the many visitors. While it was fantastic seeing all our loved ones, the long, long days were taxing. The pace was frantic but the visits were extremely gratifying.

Our days were filled with activity. Little League baseball occupied Ricky and Randy. Ricky was a full-time youth umpire while Randy was playing 2nd base in the Minors. We enjoyed the games enormously. Melissa was working part-time and preparing for her Senior year in high school. She was saving money for her first car and completing some college entrance requirements. Cheryl was a member of the Silver Lake Ski Club. Being her first year, she was very busy learning the routines of organized water skiing. Slalom water skiing was new to her but she had fun participating on a novice level. Stacey was swimming and taking piano lessons. She kept us busy just maintaining her torrid pace. Needless to say, Karen and I got involved in every one of the kids activities which we possibly could. From watching them perform to volunteering our services, we tried to be active parents. We wanted things to be "normal" for the kids. Though truthfully, they were not normal yet. I had surgery to get through and for the kids that meant mom and dad would be gone once again to Houston.

While home, the busy climate within our household was unbelievable. Karen was used to keeping these kinds of schedules — I wasn't. For me, being "Mr. Mom" was a new aspect. After two short weeks I certainly appreciated Karen's role as a housewife and mother. With the kids' schedules and activities it felt at times like we were on a short yo-yo string. They were fun, busy and TIRING days. When things got too hectic my chemoed condition left me an out, I could slip away and rest. Karen wasn't as fortunate. She would pick up my slack and run herself ragged for the kids' sake. In between all the activity, we strived to steal some private time for ourselves. It wasn't easy.

As we dealt with the day to day family occurrences my mind kept wandering towards the upcoming surgery. I was preoccupied with the prospect. A major concern for me continued to be the doctors' quandary over locating a primary site. If I was really having a rough day I'd fret about the vena cava and aorta requiring synthetic mesh to fuse them back together. When these worries began to overwhelm me I'd start saying to myself the Bible quotes I'd memorized from Dodie Osteen's *Healed of Cancer* book. More and more, I appreciated the soothing security of those special scriptures I'd chosen to lean on. More and more, I started to believe their promises. More and more, I began to feel the assurances I'd searched so hard for were contained in those simple words. Last, but not least, I understood more and more that God would have to handle it from here because I had ABSOLUTELY NO CONTROL over what happened on the operating table.

Three quotes which I repeated often throughout the day gave me the inner strength to see past all the intangibles that were looming so largely in the near future. Constantly, I reminded myself, "They worked for Dodie...why shouldn't they work for me?!"

> **"I will restore health to you, and heal you of your wounds."**
>
> *Jeremiah 30:17*

Without a doubt, health was my goal and I certainly had sustained a lot of wounds at the hands of chemotherapy and the giant tumor gnawing at my insides. Surgery was fast approaching and that would definitely be an additional big "wound" to heal from. I began to feel this scripture was written personally for me.

*****

"I shall not die, but live,
and declare the works of the Lord.
Though He has chastened me sore,
He has not given me over to death."
Psalm 118:17-18

From day one of my cancer ordeal I had no intention of submitting to cancer through death. This scripture reinforced my own attitude and exacted the singular promise to give God credit where credit was due.

*****

"Affliction will not rise up a second time."
Nahum 1:9

One of my darkest fears dwelled on getting through this immediate cancer battle...return home thinking I was fine...and suddenly face reoccurrence. Why did I think that? It was a living nightmare that I had witnessed so many times within the confines of M.D. Anderson Cancer Clinic. Even the patients who had not faced reoccurrence battled with the thought itself every time they got an ache or pain. Some admitted it, some didn't. If the truth be known, I was convinced all of us faced the thought more often than we cared to admit. From my own most apprehensive thoughts I knew that cancer was a tremendous bully! Especially if you allowed it to be! I needed, for my own peace of mind, to believe this Old Testament promise from God.

Our first week at home Karen made an appointment with our "Dearborn connection." We spent an entire morning giving blood samples in his office and waiting for the results. My blood tests all came out okay; which meant that considering chemo they were holding acceptable levels. Before we left the examination room, Logo's peer wrote prescriptions for my stomach pain and nausea. We returned home and went about our normal daily routines until the next scheduled checkup.

For me, normal routine included ignoring the pain in my stomach and tolerating some of the still clinging side effects of chemo as I tried to be a dad again. For Karen, the daily routine involved baby-sitting me, entertaining our company, and being a full-time mom again.

With the return of my appetite, I was beginning to put some weight back on my 5 foot and 11 inch frame. In the past, I'd always been a voracious eater. Being very active I'd gotten away with poor eating habits for years. From late night snacks to huge, irregular meals, I'd established bad patterns. Now, I needed to eat good food at regular intervals and in small quantities. Good nourishment fostered more strength. With surgery on the horizon, I was going to need all the strength I could put back in my depleted body. Thus, I ate and walked as often as possible.

We had been home about nine days when we received a call from M.D. Anderson tentatively scheduling my surgery for July 5, 1989. A day later we got another call from Houston. Karen took the phone call. This time it was Dr. Logothetis' office setting up tests for June 29th and 30th. Under this time frame I would have to be back in Houston by June 28th at the latest. It appeared I was going to be home for a total of seventeen days instead of the 4-5 weeks we'd counted on. This was bad enough news until Karen softly added, "Logo thinks you should have one more course of chemo...just to be sure the cancer cells are dead."

I couldn't believe my ears. Instinctively, my first response was a flat out "NO WAY!" Two major drawbacks came to my mind on the spot. If I consented to another course it would be VB4's turn. Honestly, I wasn't sure I could get through another dose of that poison. My body was still contending with side effects from the session of VB4 I had in early May. Then there was the problem of reconciling this new game plan in my own mind, since I'd been focusing all my mental energy on surgery for the last 5-6 weeks. If my mind wasn't comfortable with the newly proposed game plan it could do more harm than good. The best I could promise Karen was that I would discuss it with Logo when we returned to

Houston on June 28th.

Exercising my usual finesse, I informed Karen there would be no more trips down to the "Dearborn connection." I saw no point in wrapping up a half day in the doctor's office when in eight short days I'd be back at M.D. Anderson. Karen Marie didn't like it but she did understand where my thinking was coming from. Her conservative nature wanted me to follow the doctors' orders. My liberal attitude acknowledged the tight, new schedule thrown at us and declared the doctors' orders null and void. Even if the orders were for my own good. Smart, huh?!

The remaining days at home were spent under the dark cloud of fear and apprehension: Apprehensive of surgery and all the unknowns that go along with it. Afraid of making the wrong decision on whether or not to undergo more chemotherapy. It came down to, "What do I gain by taking more chemo?" The answer was medical reassurance. Medically, I was once more a designated statistic and statistically my chances improved. The other side of the coin was, "What do I stand to lose?" The answer was possibly my life.

My days and nights were preoccupied with these two apprehensions as the kids busy schedules continued to keep us hopping. Never was I so busy that I didn't have time to worry. Most of my concerns were kept to myself. I smiled, joked and relaxed on the surface while I fretted on the inside. True to pattern, I spoke positive or did not speak at all. And I prayed silently and often for some guidance. Karen and I seldom discussed the dilemma. With her usual common sense and loving sensitivity she knew that in the end, whatever the decision, I had to make it and be comfortable with the route chosen. My quandary was soon to be resolved.

On June 24, 1989 I received a phone call. It was early afternoon and I was alone at home. Karen and the kids were at our daughter Cheryl's ski show. Due to my forlorn appearance and the attention it drew I'd opted not to attend. I wanted to take advantage of the peace and quiet at home. With our large family it was a refreshing change because there weren't too many peaceful moments that came along during a day. I was reading when the telephone innocently rang. This phone call was the turning point for me in my battle with cancer and ALL its ugly little details.

The caller was someone I knew. A short but strange conversation ensued. When we finished talking I hung up the phone and just sat on the living room sofa thinking. I knew, without any doubt, that as far as my cancer battle went I was at the crossroads of my life. Unexplainably, I understood that it was time to make a decision. The phone call had prompted a very real awareness. The overwhelming feeling that it was time to choose between trusting myself, medicine or God. It was time to either believe what I'd been repeating to myself for almost four months...or stop saying it altogether. It was time to put up or shut up.

I knew I could go the rest of this cancer journey intact with my tough guy image and wing it alone. But, from what I'd seen with other cancer victims, I didn't like my chances or the lack of guarantees. I also knew I could trust medicine implicitly and come what may down the road. I had confidence in my doctors and had responded to treatment so far. But, there were still no concrete assurances and many who had put all their faith in medicine were now dead. They too, had responded to treatment but in the end had lost the battle to cancer. In the final tally, I would be just another statistic in someone's medical journal. I settled on God and His healing promises for my assurances. And I do mean settled.

The moment I made the mental and spiritual commitment it felt as if the weight of the whole world had been lifted from my shoulders. I really don't know if I can put the feeling into appropriate words, but here goes. In that precise moment I believed in my heart and soul that God, and his words, were the ONLY route to real peace of mind. From that moment on cancer did not scare me anymore. Surgery did not scare me. Death did not scare me. I had finally crossed the line. I had taken hope into the realm of faith. My wishes had become beliefs. It was truly exhilarating.

As the day wore on, the inner peace I'd experienced with my earlier self-commitment became more and more solidified in my mind. The peace I felt within was real and satisfying. By the time we went to bed late that Saturday night, belief in those biblical scriptures had made me as relaxed on the inside as I appeared on the outside. Karen and I fell into bed just before midnight. Somehow, I knew there would be no ugly thoughts or haunting dreams this night. In fact, I felt sure there'd be no more, period. All my suppressed fears and doubts had seemingly vanished.

At exactly 4:10 a.m. my built-in body alarm went off. The bathroom was beckoning. It was more than an urge, my bladder said it was a necessity. Early in treatment I had learned to drink lots of water during the course of a day to help flush the chemo out of my body. I glanced at our digital alarm clock as I got out of bed. Getting up in the middle of the night had become second nature to my chemoed body. Between the pain of stomach cramps and demands of my overworked bladder I'd grown accustomed to the sleeping interruptions. Tonight was different. As I was walking back to bed from the bathroom I noticed there were no cramps in my abdomen. I did not say "very little cramping" or "light cramps." I said *NONE — NO CRAMPS!* After four months of constant pain all across my lower stomach no one had to tell me the difference between some pain and *NO PAIN*. Still only half awake, I crawled back into bed wondering to myself when the pain would return.

THE HOT OIL EFFECT

Sunday, June 25, 1989 rolled in unpretentiously. By 7:30 a.m. Karen and I were out of bed, showered and ready for some breakfast. While shaving in the bathroom earlier I'd noticed the cramps were still missing. Pressing on my abdomen with my fingertips I explored all over. "Hmmmm, no pain." I wondered again when the cramps and pain would return. I hoped they wouldn't come back extra strong just to pay my body back for being absent a few hours. My daydreaming did not last long. The kids were knocking on our bedroom door like they were a hotel room service. This announced it was time to get moving.

Around 10:30 a.m. I was puttering in the living room. I bent over to pick up a magazine from the floor and put it back on the coffee table. Suddenly, it hit me. No pain! I stood bolt upright and wanted to kick myself. For the last six and one half hours I'd had no stomach pain and all I'd been able to do is wonder when the pain would return. What an idiot! I'd wished, hoped and prayed for over four months to be pain free. I'd went to bed praying and got up praying, "Please God, just take this pain from my body. Let me have some relief so I can think with no distraction." What happens? The pain decisively disappears and I don't even acknowledge the fact. Well, I did from that moment forward. I thanked God Almighty and for some reason was sure in my mind that I'd have no more stomach pain.

I casually mentioned to Karen that the cramps were gone. She was both surprised and elated. Unlike me, she didn't ask when they would be back. By noon I was outside playing baseball with Randy, Stacey and some of the neighborhood kids. A warm feeling had started to build in my lower abdomen about an hour before. At the time, I recall being only slightly aware of it. The warming trend in my body was nice but it certainly was no big deal. Not at first anyway. As the afternoon progressed the feeling became deeper and warmer. It seemed to be moving up my torso through my stomach and into my chest. Looking back, I can only say I was mindful of the growing warmth gripping my body and gradually extending upward. I really didn't understand what was going on inside my body. I just knew that it felt good. It felt calm and warm. It felt peaceful. I didn't share the feeling with anyone...I just enjoyed the inner warmth. Not until later did I realize that my body was flashing a translated message to my brain. "No pain, no cancer. No pain, no cancer." This wasn't a case of two plus two equals four. It was just a feeling. I couldn't prove it with empirical data, I could only trust the tremendous warmth that seemed to speak from within and say, "Cancer is no longer a threat to your body."

The sensation was similar to standing next to an open hearth fire on a cold, winter day and being gently warmed throughout your whole body. But it was better, much better.

It was as if someone was slowly and methodically injecting my whole body with hot oil. The penetrating warmth saturated my body inside and outside. By 7:00 p.m. that night my entire body felt aglow. I quietly wondered to myself what was going on as I continued to relish the feeling and went about my usual business.

When we got into bed after midnight the warmth was still present. Laying there in bed, next to Karen Marie, the notion remained with me that I was not contaminated by cancer anymore. I was certain that the cancer in my body was completely dead. In fact, I wasn't too sure there was any cancer — dead or alive — left in my body. I felt cleansed and completely healed. The feeling came from deep within. It was not a conclusion my mind arrived at...it was just an intense FEELING of real knowledge. The sensation was as real as the bed under me. It was unexplainable but even more it was undeniable.

For the first time in over a year I slept on my stomach. Awaking Monday morning I was immediately aware that the intense, glowing warmth was gone. But the knowledge of "*no cancer*" which had been manifested by yesterday's inner glow remained. I felt absolutely positive that all cancer was dead and/or gone. This presented a dilemma.

How do I share a feeling with someone and tell them that without a doubt I know it to be a fact? I mean, a fact is a fact and a feeling is just that...a feeling. A fact is something you can see and understand; a feeling is something you cannot see and not always understand. One is tangible and credible; the other is intangible and incredible. To me the whole episode was [in]credible. Pun intended.

The experience was mine alone. I don't expect others to understand something they did not personally experience but I do expect others to accept the possibility of the experience. In more ways than one, the validity of my "feeling" would be resolved with surgery.

Time was winding down for me at home. I had to be back in Houston for two days of testing by June 28, 1989. Karen and I agreed that I should go back alone while she would remain at home for a few extra days. We felt the abbreviated recovery time was hard enough for me to accept...there was no sense in Karen and the kids being punished by the change in schedule. Remember, we had originally told the kids we would be home for at least a month prior to surgery. They were banking on those words and seventeen (17) days do not make a month. The revised plan was that Karen would follow me to Houston in a few more days.

THE CLIMAX of SURGERY

At noon, on June 28th I landed at Houston Hobby Airport. As usual, I missed Karen Marie. Her physical presence was always a reassuring blanket of protection. She was my emotional bodyguard and I missed her being at my side. It was hot, hot, hot as I waited for a shuttle bus. The humidity was 100 percent and the temperature was 91 degrees. The air felt as if I were in a sauna.

The controversy concerning surgery versus more chemotherapy was much on my mind. I'd made my decision. Come *Hell* or high water, I was going to follow my "feeling." My game plan was to stick with the scheduled surgery; and no more chemo! Now, all I had to do was convince Logo. I knew this would not be easy because Logo was cautious. More chemo was a mandatory safeguard to him. To me it was unnecessary. I grabbed a shuttle bus and went directly to our Houston apartment. From there, I dropped my luggage and went straight to the Lutheran Building [the hospital wing] to locate Dr. Logothetis.

When I got to the M.D. Anderson complex it was bristling with energetic bodies. Took me more than an hour to run Logo down and see if he could fit me in for an unscheduled conference. I knew he'd make time for our confab whether he had it to spare or not. That was the way Dr. Logothetis operated. He believed in treating the mental and emotional roadblocks of a patient before you began treating the patient physically. Many in the medical profession could take a lesson from his standard operating procedure. If you think about it, Logo's method just made good common sense. It amounted to addressing the patient's fears and reservations prior to any kind of actual medical treatment.

During our discussion, I opted for the July 5, 1989 scheduled surgery which was only seven days away. He opted for more chemotherapy and postponing surgery. From past experience, I knew Logo could be very persuasive and convincing in his arguments. He firmly believed that more chemo was in my best interests. On the other hand, I was committed to the feeling that I did not need more chemotherapy. We agreed to weigh each other's side and think it over until the next day.

When I left Logo's office I started up to the ninth floor to see if any of my friends were in treatment. On the elevator, I ran into Pat "M" and his fiance, Judy. Their home state was South Dakota. Pat was pulling an I.V. cart with chemo bags and antibiotics dangling from it. He was hoping to finish this dose of chemo, make a trip home for a little while and then return to Houston for the remainder of his treatment. Stepping out of the elevator we continued talking as I followed them outside to enjoy some sunshine and fresh air.

Pat had been in treatment for a long time. He was another testicular non-seminoma patient. An obvious tumor was being treated in the left side of his neck. Distressingly, complications from chemotherapy seemed to be continually delaying his treatments. The setbacks were understandably hard on Pat's attitude. Though overall, he was doing as good as he possibly could battling the emotional strains of cancer.

Despite Pat and Judy keeping pretty much to themselves in his 9th floor room, Karen and I had met them last month. Just before our trip home to rest up for surgery we'd encountered them in the Lutheran building lobby. Karen and Judy had liked each other immediately. Like Karen, she was very supportive. And like Karen and me, they made a warm, loving couple. They were a team in their struggle against Pat's cancer. I enjoyed seeing them and shooting the breeze for awhile. Wrapped up our visit by telling them Karen would be with me next week and we'd look them up after I was admitted.

As I waited for a shuttle back to our apartment my thoughts were preoccupied with Pat. I'd been around M.D. Anderson Cancer Clinic long enough to know that Pat's prognosis did not appear real good. From what I'd been witness to with other patients, I reasoned that if the tumor was in his neck then it must have travelled the whole lymph node system to arrive there. That's a long journey from the primary site in the testicles and did not paint a very pretty picture. Getting on the shuttle bus, I wondered if he was aware of the implications. From what I saw in his eyes, I think he had an idea of the growing graveness. His eyes held the same fear and panic which I'd seen in so many other eyes down here. Cancer had a way of doing that to you.

On Friday, June 30th, I bumped into Logo in front of the Lutheran Building entrance. I'd completed my series of tests and was waiting for the Brompton Apartment's shuttle bus. It was in the afternoon and Logo was returning to the hospital. He asked if I had a few minutes and I answered in the affirmative. Up to his 7th floor office we went. Once there, he sat me down and we talked for a long time. We both had our say. Our conversation centered on medicine and statistics from Logo's point of view; my side was not so easily supported. It was based strictly on a feeling. In the end, Logo consented to the soon scheduled surgery. The only stipulation being that if there was even a hint of live cancer cells discovered in my body during the operation he would ask the surgeons to immediately close me back up. That would mean more chemo. I agreed.

Then, and now, I realize Logo had my best interests at heart. But, so did I! To me, surgery was not a gamble. To Logo, it was statistically an immense gamble. Without mincing words, he felt surgery at that point was just plain stupid. I didn't expect him to understand where I was coming from. The feeling that my body was void of cancer was solely mine. The experience which led me to that conviction was uniquely mine. It was my body and my life and I knew inherently that what I felt inside was accurate. There was not a doubt in my heart that the tumor was dead and there was no live cancer anywhere in my body. And I mean not a doubt.

After leaving Logo's office I was relieved that the pitched battle of words was out of the way and put to rest. The decision had been made and that gave me some real peace of mind. Plus, I had something to look forward to; Karen Marie would be flying back into Houston on July 3rd. Admittedly, I was just plain lonesome and anxious for her return. With surgery firmly set for Wednesday, July 5th, it was time to get the final stage of this show on the road. I figured with chemotherapy behind me the worst was over. In my mind, surgery would be a breeze compared to chemo and its side effects. Only one small detail was overlooked. I'd forgotten to take into account that *I WAS NOT IN CHARGE* of this healing show. Unfortunately, recovery from surgery would soon refresh my memory.

I picked Karen up from Houston Hobby Airport on July 3, 1989. She was a sight to behold. Her casual beauty made my temperature rise. It was a shame but we had very little time to cherish our reunion. Unbeknownst to Karen, we were on a very tight schedule. In itself, this was certainly nothing new for either of us! I had been late picking her up at the airport because I still wasn't admitted to the hospital. In fact, I'd waited for almost two hours in the admissions office and had to leave for the airport just as my turn arrived.

We utilized the driving time back to M.D. Anderson to exchange information. I brought Karen up to date on all the events which had taken place down here in her absence. In turn, she brought me up to date on our kids and events back home. Karen was most concerned over my discussion with Logo. Upon hearing the highlights she became very quiet. After 18 years of marriage I knew she had to reconcile this new information in her own mind and then she'd be fine. Although she made it clear she did not agree with the surgery decision, Karen staunchly stood by me once she realized my conviction. In my heart, I'd known she would.

The admissions office closed at 5:00 p.m. and it was already 4:30 p.m. so we were cutting it close. I had to be officially admitted that afternoon because the next day was the fourth of July and the hospital administrative offices would be closed. The plan was to be admitted on paper and assigned a room on the 6th floor even though we didn't have to be bodily there until July 4th. It was close but we made it. Finally, all the pre-surgery arrangements appeared to be in motion.

Also on July 3rd, my dad and mom, Rick and Ella Rockman, were coming into Houston by train. Their arrival had been firmly set for a week. They were worried about me and insisted on being present for the upcoming surgery. Actually, dad and mom had boarded the train in Michigan for the three day trip to Houston knowing that my surgery was an unsettled point of controversy. Now that all systems were "go" I was glad they would be here to give Karen some much needed support during the operation. We picked them up from the Amtrak station about 9:00 p.m. that night. What the long train ride didn't drain from them the Houston heat and humidity did. They were worn out. When I saw how tired they looked I couldn't help but harass my dad just a little about being afraid to fly. After almost 1600 miles by train I think at that moment he may have reconsidered and taken a plane. Then again, I'm not too sure.

Karen and I celebrated the 1989 fourth of July by checking into a private room on the 6th floor of M.D. Anderson hospital. We felt right at home. It had only been about three weeks since our last hospital stay. By 9:30 a.m. we were settled in room 6036 and awaiting doctors' orders. My dad and mom were unpacked and just as settled back at our apartment. The apartment would be conveniently theirs for the next week or more so we wanted them to make themselves at home. Karen would be staying in the hospital with me as she always did. Because of this fact, I've nominated her for a *best supporting spouse Oscar* for sleeping in a foldout chair most of the last five months and "acting" like it was a real bed. She gets my vote for best supporting wife with no complaints. She also gets my vote for deepest devotion to a cause. And that cause was plainly ME.

On this particular fourth of July, the only fireworks we viewed were on television. Karen's fondness for holidays elicited a promise from me to make it up to her next year with an extra special July 4th celebration. I had every intention of keeping that verbal promise.

July 5, 1989 dawned like most other summer Texas days. Houston was poised for another hot, humid day. The temperature was forecast in the mid 90 degree range and the stifling humidity would be up around 100 percent. Just as naturally, Karen and I woke up in the confines of M.D. Anderson as we had so often in the last five months. The only obvious difference was that I was in the hospital for major surgery instead of chemotherapy.

At long last, the climax of this cancer struggle was imminent. I was ready for surgery. We'd been five long months anticipating this day. The tumor, or what was left of it, was going to be removed. The filthy contamination that I'd felt and lived with for months was going to be lifted via the surgeon's scalpel. I was relaxed, optimistic and calm. The peace which I'd discovered just a week ago was very evident. It was not a front or a bunch of false bravado. It was genuine peace of mind.

Sometime after 12:00 noon orderlies wheeled me down to the 4th floor pre-op waiting room on a surgical stretcher. I'd said good-bye to my dad and mom back in our room and Karen had escorted me the rest of the way. We talked and fondly kidded while waiting for my turn in the operating room. Karen was one big, loving smile as we waited. She knew in her heart every single area of concern was going to turn out alright. All I did was verbally reinforce those feelings for her. Her reservoir of inner strength truly amazed me. Looking back, maybe I was a little too calm that day because I never did receive the pre-op relaxation shot which I'd expected. With a last teary-eyed embrace from Karen the nurse announced it was time for my surgery. Off to the OR [Operating Room] I went. It was 1:00 p.m., July 5, 1989 when I was eventually positioned on the operating table. I remember my impression vividly, "*This table is cold, very cold.*" The OR atmosphere was quiet and very business like. One of the attending nurses asked if I was alright. "I'm ready to roll," was my reply. The anesthesiologist was the last person I recall seeing before the lights went out. My lights that is.

The next thing I was aware of was feeling wrapped up like

a mummy and hearing a familiar voice. It was Logo. He was gently touching my leg as he quietly said, "You were right, Richard...everything went fine. All we're waiting for is the pathology report." I tried to smile. Instead, I rasped out, "Where's Karen?" Logo replied, "You're not supposed to have visitors in here...let me see what I can do."

I was in post-op. This is an intensive care recovery room which closely monitors a patient for the critical few hours following major surgery. The operation had taken six hours and 20 minutes. Squinting through a small opening, my eyes immediately gathered that I was bound with tape and gauze from the top of my head down to my groin. Groggily, I tried to regain the rest of my senses. My mind was clear enough to remember to thank God for confirming with surgery what only I had known — the cancer in my body had been dead and now was gone.

I'd awakened with plenty of discomfort and was beginning to feel pain. My whole body seemed to ache. The inside of my throat felt as if it had been scraped raw with rough sandpaper. Something in the right side of my neck hurt and at the same time prevented me from being able to move my head much. Later I found out that this was a large I.V. needle put in during the operation as a precaution. If an emergency blood transfusion were necessary, this neck site would be available. My arms felt as if they were strapped down and out to my side. I could see an I.V. line coming from both of my hands. They throbbed like a toothache. Then I felt the catheter pull as I tried to flex my legs and turn on my side. I thought to myself, "Why do I have one of those stupid things in me?" No one had told me I would be bound and gagged like King Tut after surgery! I was getting frustrated and angry until I heard Karen's soothing voice. "It's all over, Rick."

Peering from beneath the bandages I could see her shadowy figure standing there, at my side. Honest to God, she looked like an angel as my eyes focused on her. The relieved smile on her face made me feel warm all over. I think my first words to Karen were, "I missed you." Then I proceeded to whisper in a gravelly voice, "What's all this stuff on me?" She sensed I was getting agitated and worked up. She held my hand and tried to explain all the restraining articles around my body. Trusting the comfort of her touch, I closed my eyes and listened through all the bandages and paraphernalia surrounding me. Just the sound of her reassuring voice settled me down. After a few minutes, the 2nd shift nurse reminded Karen it was time to leave. Vaguely, I remember telling her that I didn't want her to go. She stayed a little longer and then carefully leaned over and kissed me saying, "Honey, I have to go now...your mom and dad are waiting. We'll see you in the morning. Get some rest...I love you."

Thanks to some genuine inner peace I had not worried about all the intangibles of surgery. I'd found peace and strength by letting God handle those intangibles. I can honestly state I was totally relaxed at the prospect of surgery. It not only hadn't frightened or intimidated me, I had actually looked forward to the event. First of all, I'd wanted to get it over with and placed in the past along with a lot of other painful episodes which cancer introduced. Second, the only way the doctors were going to believe that my body was cancer free was to have it medically substantiated. Surgery and the clean pathology report had confirmed that point.

When the surgeons opened me up, all that had remained of the original, huge tumor was a well-defined dead mass. The mass was the size, shape and consistency of an over baked potato when the surgeons removed its deadened remains on July 5th. This was a far cry from the 7 inch x 18 inch active malignancy which had been present a short few months ago. The aorta and vena cava which I'd worried so much about in the past, survived surgery virtually unscathed. Amazingly, these large veins were left intact with no permanent damage sustained by penetration of the tumor. The area surrounding the aorta and vena cava had demanded some very meticulous work by the surgeons but had required no fusing or rebuilding with synthetic mesh. Tediously, the team of surgeons had spent hours scraping the tumor's dead particles from around my spine. After all the complications and heartbreak I'd witnessed at the expense of other patients at M.D. Anderson I considered myself extremely fortunate. No one had to remind me to count my blessings! I thanked

God for answering ALL my prayers. Specifically, I thanked God for my loving wife, Karen Marie and our healthy children. Then, I thanked God for leading us to these doctors and this cancer facility.

THE ANTI-CLIMAX of RECOVERY

In some ways surgery was the easiest part of my cancer journey. In other ways it was the most difficult. Surgery was the easiest part of my journey because the doctors did the brunt of the work. They painstakingly removed what was left of the malignant tumor and its intruding tentacles. In laymen's terms, they delicately strip-mined my abdominal lymph node system in the process. The doctors also took sample tissue from various areas surrounding the tumor and routinely sent it to pathology for analysis. ALL tissue had to be completely free of live cancer cells to receive a medical thumbs up. That was the desired result and foremost reason for the intense chemotherapy I underwent. M.D. Anderson's surgery team, headed by Dr. Kenneth Wishnow, had done an excellent job. The only "apparent" work they left for me was recovering from the vertical 12 inch incision they made which ran from my groin to just below my rib cage. It extended right down the middle of my body with an "S" curve at the belly button. Following surgery, I regretfully discovered my body had much more to recover from than just that large incision.

In retrospect, the main reason that surgery ended up being so very difficult came from my own mouth and mind. First of all, I had it in my head that this surgery, and the subsequent recovery period, would be like any others I had previously experienced. Through the years, I'd been operated on seven different times for everything from a hernia and knee repair to an appendectomy and bone grafts. I was under the mistaken impression that I was well-acquainted with all the aspects of surgery and recovery. The doctors would do the surgical repairing and I would do the physical recuperating. At least, that's how the situation laid out in *my* mind.

From past practice, I never babied myself after surgery. I'd always stayed active and pushed my body to respond to its natural healing process with food, water, exercise and fresh air. I tried to use the same regimen this time and it spelled disaster. To start with, I wasn't allowed ANY food or water. Furthermore, I would not be allowed any food or water until my bowels showed signs of functioning. No food meant no nourishment. No water meant possible dehydration. No liquid or solid nourishment meant no recovery strength. It added up to an imposed starvation diet.

The radical lymph node dissection I'd undergone was much more involved than any of my prior experiences with the surgeon's scalpel. My internal organs had been moved, jostled and just plain messed with during the long, involved surgery. To enhance a clear view and clean path to the tumor site, the surgeons had actually set some of my internal organs outside my body for hours during the operation. Over one hundred surgical hemaclips [small metal clips which resemble a staple] were used to tie off the small blood vessels which had been disrupted during the scraping away of dead cancer cells around my spine and within my abdomen. Also, a drainage tube for my stomach was inserted during surgery. The need for hemaclips and this protruding plastic tube supported the reality of my internal organs' disruption. The hemaclips were a permanent addition to my internal anatomy while the plastic tube was a temporary fixture.

Even though I recognized the temporary aggravation, I hated that tube more than anything else. It came to symbolize the way I underestimated surgery and recovery because I could not go home until that drainage tube was removed. Frustratingly, the plain medical facts were: the tube would not be removed until my bowels and digestive system were operating. It was like a jigsaw puzzle—my internal organs were the separate pieces and yet they were all connected parts of the whole. Thus, my body couldn't move on to another phase of recovery until the first phase fell into place.

Trying to take control again, I leaned even more on the

PAR I'd established during chemo treatment, with the emphasis on prayer. Unconsciously, I tried to hurry God's plan of healing and rush the natural mending power of the body because it fit*my* needs and desires. This attempt to once more take control of the situation eventually spelled disaster.

Everyday after surgery, during his morning rounds, I would ask Dr. Scott Hassell [a Fellowship surgeon] to remove the drainage tube. Everyday he would patiently explain that it could not be removed until my internal organs started to function. He was dealing *with* reality, while I was dealing *out* wishful thinking. On some of those mornings it must have occurred to Dr. Hassell that I took his last name literally because each day seemed to start with a mild "hassle" over when I was going home to Michigan. Evidently, Dr. Hassell wasn't aware of the promise I'd made to our 15 year old daughter!

In addition to thinking recovery would be a snap and proceed according to *my* expectations, I'd compounded the erroneous thoughts by also running off at the mouth. Before coming back to Houston for surgery I told our second oldest daughter (Cheryl), that we'd be home in time to celebrate her 16th birthday with her. That would be July 19th, only two weeks to the day after undergoing surgery.

Honestly, my purpose when making the promise was no more than utilizing continued positive thinking. Plus, I just as honestly felt that two weeks was plenty of time to recover from ANY operation. It turned out to be an error in judgement. I had confused reality with wishful thinking. My past surgery experiences had left some unrealistic ideas as they pertained to this radical procedure. I believed my own words when I made the ill-fated promise to our daughter but it sure didn't turn out that way. No food or water was the doctors' order of the day and my Achilles heel. When July 19th rolled around, ice chips [and I had to sneak those] were the closest thing to food which entered my mouth in the fourteen days directly following surgery.

Two other people were also unaware of the promise I'd made to Cheryl. They were my longtime and close friends, Carl and Ben, who had grown up and went to school with me in little old Fenton. I had been so sure that recovery would proceed on *my* premature schedule that I'd arranged to have our car driven from Texas to Michigan. Imposing on our friendship, I'd asked Carl and Ben if they would fly out to Houston and drive our car back home. Ideally, they would be chauffeuring the car and some of our personal belongings for the long return trip. My plan was that Carl and Ben would get the car back to Michigan prior to July 19, 1989 so Karen and I would have transportation when we arrived home. Like the true friends they are they graciously accepted without hesitation. As it turned out, Carl and Ben lived up to their end of the commitment — mine was another story.

Before you can digest food you have to be sure your body can remove that same food. At this point, mine couldn't. To help myself towards recovery, about the only thing I could do was walk. With great effort, I walked and walked. The large incision and my insides being torn up made me move like a ninety year old man. In my weakened condition, the walks exhausted what little energy I possessed. My bowels, bladder and intestines were not fully functioning. In fact, they seemed to be barely functioning at all. With each day of imposed fasting I was becoming more and more dehydrated.

The lack of nourishment from not eating was beginning to show on me emotionally as well as physically. In Karen's words it came out like this: "Rick, you are nutritionally starved. You're not acting like yourself." The doctors agreed with Karen. They decided I needed hyperalimentation instead of waiting for my body to accept natural food and water intake. This decision presented a problem. My veins were too distended from the past chemo and recent surgery to accommodate the thick, liquid nourishment through a regular I.V. line. Thus, before I could receive the hyper-al it was going to be necessary to insert another CVC line. More grief for me because my tolerance for needles and incisions was about zero at this point. Eventually, I listened to Karen and the medical consensus as I relented to the CVC line being implanted beneath my right collarbone. Once more, I found out the hard way that just because I desired something did not mean it was going to happen. I'd had my heart and mind set

on going home as soon as possible but it was not to be. Karen
continually reminded me that recovery would take time, a lot
of time. Nobody knew how much.

Surgery was the last step on the journey home. It represented the climax to months of tribulation. The recovery from
surgery ended up being the anti-climax. I had done my part.
I'd been as tough and durable as possible through chemotherapy and surgery. The doctors had done their part.
Through treatment and surgery they had been compassionate and professionally adept. The medicine had even done its
part. Though I admit this with a deep reluctance to call chemo
drugs medicine. Poison remains my favorite term of description. Now, just plain old "time" had to do its part in the
healing process. If I could be patient enough to let it!

Recovery from surgery was an anti-climax for which I had
not prepared. I had thought that with the culmination of
surgery my marathon race was finished. Was I ever wrong!
By analogy, I still had miles to go when I ran into "the wall."
A wall called recovery time. Due to my own short-sighted
recovery goals and usual impatience, the PAR which I'd used
so successfully in the recent past wasn't enough. I didn't
forget God was my ally but I was caught up in asking prayers
to supersede the body's natural healing process. I seemed to
forget that God had provided for healing with just the
creative design of our anatomy. Humbly, I learned that the
mending process of the human body had its own plan for
recovery time. One more instance of comprehending that my
willpower did not control the situation. My impatience and
unrealistic appraisal of recovery time almost did me in.
Literally.

On July 26, 1989, exactly three weeks after surgery, Karen
and I were back in Michigan. Against their better judgement,
my Houston doctors had removed the drainage tube and
newly implanted CVC line to allow my release from M.D.
Anderson Hospital. Maybe I wore them down arguing about
going home. I guess we'll never know for sure. As it turned
out, I won the battle to go home but I lost the war to a speedy
recovery.

On July 28, 1989, exactly three weeks and two days after

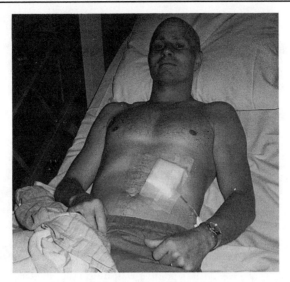

Immediately following surgery, about July 8, 1989.

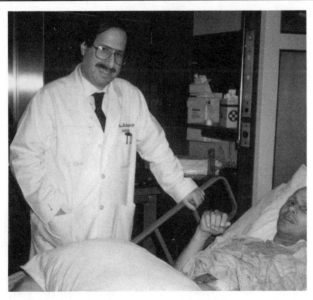

Dr. Kenneth Wishnow, my surgeon, making a post-op checkup.

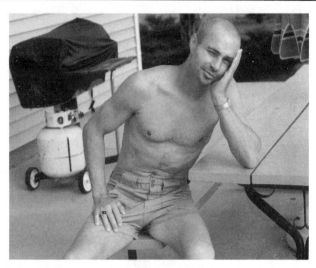

Labor Day 1989. At this point, I was anticipating better days ahead and feeling as weak as I looked.

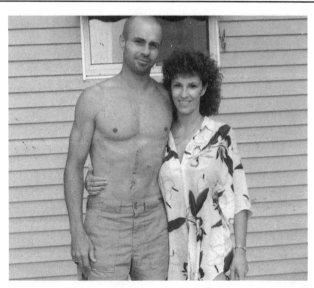

Another Labor Day 1989 picture. Karen and I pose on the patio in our backyard with me still gaunt and still hurting.

surgery, I was back in the hospital — a Michigan hospital this time. Our final homecoming was marred by my impatience. Soon after returning home I tried to eat solid food. More than anything else, I felt my body needed real nourishment and my mind needed to know my body was getting *REAL* nourishment. And I didn't mean popsicles and jello!

Ignorantly, on our second day home, I attempted to digest a piece of pizza [with double cheese no less] and my body was nowhere near ready for this type of solid food. My diet was supposed to be tiny quantities of soup, crackers and baby food. I paid dearly for the deviation from soft foods. Very quickly, and in a very big way, I became deathly sick. Terrible stomach cramps and fever set in. There was so much pressure that the large incision that ran the length of my abdomen felt as if it was going to split wide open. Karen loaded me up and headed for the hospital.

We spent four, miserable, pain-filled hours in the Flint Osteopathic Hospital [FOH] emergency room. Upon admission to FOH, where my cancer saga had begun almost 6 months earlier, I was completely dehydrated. Even my brain was nutritionally starved at this point. As in Houston, I couldn't think clearly or maintain my balance. Because of dehydration my emotions were about skin deep at best. Simply put, I was a mess when we arrived at FOH emergency. Our family physician, Dr. Robert Hamilton, immediately started me on intravenous sugar water to combat the dehydration. The attending doctors were concerned that I had acute ileitis [inflammation of the opening at bottom of small intestines] or a bowel obstruction. The hospital routine was once again wait, watch and listen.

The I.V. feeding did its desired work. My body's dehydrated condition was being slowly reversed. Soon, I felt almost human again. At least I could carry on a conversation and walk with marginal balance. I'd been on the liquid food for about 48 hours when in the early morning of my third day at FOH I contacted my doctor by phone. As politely as possible, I informed him that regardless of the consequences I had to get out of this hospital environment. I did my best to explain that the hospital atmosphere was having a negative impact on the chances for my body to recover from surgery. I was prepared to saddle up and just walk out but Dr. Hamilton graciously consented to officially discharging me. He recognized the symptoms of medical phobia I guess. I'd reached my limit for doctors, nurses, tests and needles. At this point, I felt the mental drawbacks of the hospital far outweighed the physical drawbacks I might experience at home. On July 30, 1989 I walked out of Flint Osteopathic Hospital. Slowly staggered might be more accurate. Anyway, home I went.

When I returned home this time I took it easy. As Karen Marie reminded me, I had no choice. My body was a mess. For some curious reason the side effects associated with chemotherapy appeared to escalate after surgery. It seemed the weaker I became, the more some of my old chemo side effects would manifest themselves. My weight was down to less than 128 pounds. How much less we'll never know because I had quit getting on the scales a week prior, while still in Houston. The tale of the scales had become downright depressing. There was not a hair left on my body. Not just my head, mind you, but my whole body. It appeared I'd be going through puberty twice in one lifetime. There was no muscle tone *IN my body* because there was no muscle anywhere *ON my body*. I was skin and bones. I virtually looked like a concentration camp survivor.

My left leg and arm continued to go numb periodically and throb with pain. This, and the complete hair loss, were evidently lingering side effects of chemotherapy. Realizing the chemo holdovers, I knew I had to be extremely careful of pneumonia. From observing other patients' misfortunes I was well aware that a weakened body is susceptible to pneumonia. I was just as aware that pneumonia kills. To combat the pneumonia I forced myself to do deep breathing exercises at least four times a day and continued walking. Pneumonia and ANY Intensive Care Unit were two areas of grief which I was bound and determined to avoid.

My physical weakness eventually wore my emotions down. It was an hourly battle to think positive and envision myself whole and healthy again. If you recall, I've already stated my opinion that body weakness promotes fear and frustration. It harbors doubts and plays negatively on your mind. I was no exception to this opinion. Sometimes, even being aware of this stumbling block was not enough to overcome the depression. I could not eat yet. My body and brain were still being nutritionally starved because my digestive system had not begun to fully function. No real food meant that I was going to continue to battle physical weakness and emotional weariness. Suffice to say, even with my daily PAR, it was difficult to see a silver lining in this cloud.

To our kids way of thinking, I was home therefore I must be okay. A logical conclusion on their part but a false premise. I had no strength, no energy and no stamina. Resuming the regular pace of our daily lives was a tremendous adjustment for both Karen and myself. Physically, mentally and emotionally it was demanding. There was nothing wrong with my nose or appetite and this made my inability to eat solid foods even harder to accept. Smelling the delicious odors coming from our kitchen each evening was a real problem. We would sit down as a family and have our dinner with me sipping soup broth and the rest of the family enjoying Karen's delectable cooking. It played on my mind after awhile. Dealing with phones, visitors and schedules each day would zap what little strength I had left. By the end of a normal day I was totally drained.

On August 4th, the battle of recovery culminated with a bad night. Around 9:30 p.m. that Friday night, I retreated to our bedroom to lie down. Stretched out on the bed and staring at the ceiling tears suddenly welled up in my eyes. My body and mind were in a miserable state. Recovery from surgery had become one long nightmare. The same thoughts kept running through my head. *How can I try so hard to feel well and feel so utterly bad? What's wrong with me?...What am I doing wrong?* I began to sob softly. Karen, with her usual intuition and timing, found me shortly with the tears now quietly trickling down my cheeks.

She came over to our king-size bed, laid down next to me and held my head and face in her arms. "It's going to be alright, it's going to be alright...trust me...I know it is," she whispered.

"I don't know how much more I can take," angrily I spat it out. "I can't eat. I can't think. I can hardly walk...I wish someone would put a .357 to my head and pull the trigger. Just put me out of my misery." The words rolled out of my mouth. I really don't know where the thought which prompted those words came from, but I do know that I said them. The selfish, depressed comment hurt and surprised Karen. To tell the truth it surprised me. I knew that I didn't walk around all day and think those negative ideas. Yet, it had popped out of my mouth.

Karen replied, "You don't mean that. You're just frustrated and weak. You'll feel better if you have a good cry...if you let your tears go all the way. Quit holding back." She stroked my face with her hands and let my comment pass with a final resolute remark, "We've come too far to give in now."

I listened, but said nothing. I understood that feeling sorry for myself was self-destructive...yet, the frustration of not being able to eat, coupled with the depression of weakness had become overwhelming. Ironically, voicing those self-pitying words took the edge off my seemingly uncontrollable emotions. I felt better now that the verbal vomit was out. I was tired, very tired.

Before leaving me to myself, Karen sat up over me and looked me straight in the eyes as she reminded me one more time, "Rick, you expect too much, too quick. You have been through Hell. Your mind and body are literally starved for nutrition. Until you start eating again your mind and body are not going to function as you want them to. Be patient, Honey. *You* have to be patient."

I slept the sleep of the dead that night. My body never moved until our alarm sounded at 5:15 a.m. the next morning. This announced it was time to get Ricky up for his newspaper job. I'd volunteered the afternoon before to take him into work. My body still looked wretched but inside I felt better. Though still extremely weak, my spirits were back on an even keel. I sipped soup broth that morning for breakfast, kept it down and then hoped my body could handle the other end of the eating cycle...expelling it.

Sometimes you have to hit bottom before you can start back towards the top. That's exactly what happened with me. I wasted very little energy with self-condemnation or personal reproach. Guilt was not allowed to shadow me over these low points. In my mind, the incident of the night before was no more than a temporary setback. Actually, in itself, it served as a catalyst. I began once again to count my blessings instead of counting my hurts. It was a confident, warm feeling to be back on track. Karen Marie reminded me often to let God's masterful design of the human body take care of the recovery process. In other words — *be patient!*

On Sunday, August 6, 1989 we had two great causes for celebration. Number one: it was Karen's 39th birthday. Number two: I ate my first real solid meal in over a month. The kids and I took Karen Marie out for breakfast and I had an omelette, toast and juice.

How did I know it was time to try solid food? I didn't know. Not for certain, anyway. Without setting goals this time, I used the same PAR which had led me through many other difficult circumstances. I prayed, positive imaged and walked in anticipation of eating once again. To make a long story short I just felt that it was time to eat again. The feeling wasn't strictly from hunger pains, it was just a convincing calm feeling that my body would accommodate food now. I'd listened to strictly hunger pains nine days back and ended up in the hospital. This time I listened to God's peaceful direction within my inner senses. It worked.

From the date of Karen's birthday and forward, my eating habits began to return to normal. By the end of September '89 I was beginning to feel human again. After enduring six months of intense chemotherapy, major surgery and the ensuing recovery period, the rainbow I had pursued so diligently was arcing brighter each day. My body was progressively gaining weight. Some muscle tone was creeping back into my arms and legs in conjunction with the weight gain. Even my bald head and body were beginning to sprout hair once again.

All in all, my life, Karen's, and the kids' was getting back on track. Our lives were slowly, but surely, assuming gradual degrees of normalcy. It was a huge adjustment period for all concerned.

As before, Karen and I had to reestablish our authority and the kids had to find security in our presence. Mutual love and respect were the passwords of the day in our home. They had to be as we tried not to live in the past. Instead, we conveyed to the kids that this was a fresh start; what was done was done. I remember looking around the room at all their faces as we had a family meeting to air some problems and hear some of their complaints. What I saw was three very impressionable teenagers, one teenager in training [our 11 year old], and the youngest [our 9 year old], who was soon to be a teenager in training. Their suspicious expressions said it all; the turmoil of my cancer struggle had hurt them too. Our imposed exodus to Houston for six months had left them scarred with doubt and insecurity. Karen and I agreed, they were just trying to grow into young adults and my cancer had interrupted the natural transition. Undeniably, the teen years are tough on kids and parents alike — WITHOUT dealing with the likes of cancer. Other than periodic checkups back in Houston, we promised them that we were home to stay. This statement was the starting point to regaining their trust and confidence.

Our children were not the only ones adapting to change. Both of us had to adapt to many circumstances for which we were not prepared. One area we learned to get used to was the fact that neither of us was ever allowed to put cancer in our past for any length of time. We were constantly running into someone who had not seen us since our return home. This almost always prompted a conversation about cancer and my long range medical prognosis. When our friends and acquaintances heard from our lips that I was fine, thanks to God and medicine, most flashed a look of disbelief. Many thought I was in remission and had a difficult time comprehending that we believed I was cured of cancer and healed forever. These were basically the same people who had said prayers, sent cards and offered assistance while we were in Houston, Texas.

Armed with this knowledge, Karen and I used patience and understanding to combat some of the poorly disguised doubt. We understood their uncertain stares because we realized better than anybody that there were very few happy endings with cancer. Time will take care of the doubt. Until then, we enjoy the sincere concern of all these people. They were a real support system and we appreciated them from the bottom of our hearts.

Chapter 10

THE FINAL ANALYSIS

It's been a long haul getting to this point but we're finally here. In all honesty, a person could probably read the introduction of this book and then skip right to this last chapter to discover the message I've diligently attempted to deliver. But, you'd be missing one very important factor. Credibility! To get my message across to present and future cancer victims I felt strongly that you needed to understand how and why I came to my conclusions. The credibility is based on my personal experience in battling cancer. Circumstances, people and feelings made the experience.

You read about my cancer struggle as I lived it — one step at a time — one day at a time. Through nine chapters you have battled cancer emotionally, physically and financially right alongside me. You have undergone chemotherapy and surgery. You have struggled against the futile feelings of helplessness and hopelessness. You have searched for assurances and guarantees that were not available. You have labored through financial hardship. In essence, you have taken a faith walk with me. All that remains is the lessons learned. *You* are the reason I gave over six months of my life to writing a saga that might have been better personally to leave in the past. By that I mean I did not need to write this story for my benefit...I'd already lived it.

SOMETHING to OFFER

Drawn from my own experience and what I've witnessed on a daily basis as I come in contact with other patients, the dominant response to initial cancer detection appears to be an overwhelming *FEAR of the UNKNOWN*. Fear of a word associated exclusively with pain, grief and death. Fear of a disease called cancer and the medical treatments utilized against it.

Unless you have personally heard the mental death sentence which cancer brings you cannot envision the emotional despair. Upon hearing the words, "I'm sorry, you have cancer," your earthly existence suddenly becomes very fragile. It brings with it the stark realization that you no longer have control over your own future. Your destiny is in someone else's hands. The cancer victim is abruptly thrown into a world measured by degrees of grief. When the medical verdict comes in it has three unofficial interpretations. ONE: Your type of cancer is treatable — mankind has remedies. There is medical hope. TWO: Your type of cancer is treatable but not beatable — mankind has temporary remedies which may prolong your life. There is some help but little long range medical hope. THREE: Your type of cancer is not treatable — mankind has no known remedy. There is no medical hope.

No matter which heading you may fall under, the truth is that you immediately cease to be a person. Instead you become a medical statistic. Cancer steals your identity as a real live human being and relegates you to a plus or minus on the survival chart. This is where cancer begins to establish its grip on you. This is the point where cancer emotionally starts to manhandle you: *If you allow it*. This is also the point you need to know exactly what you are up against. You need to understand that what you are facing is truly a life or death situation and that the outcome is extremely personal. It does not get any more personal than fighting for your life!

These are candid observations; views that were not drawn solely from my own struggle with cancer. More than an opinion, I'm offering impressions left by the experiences of other cancer victims which I see repeated over and over in the hospitals. I'm offering insight drawn from the many phone conversations with other cancer victims who have contacted us at our home. From all across the United States they call wanting one thing...HELP in battling cancer. These people

want to know *what* to do and *how* to do it! They are scared and
bewildered. Collectively, they are as lost and helpless as
Karen and I were back in February of 1989.

This kind of frankness paints a dark picture but please
don't throw in the towel yet. Don't give in to these sometimes
overwhelming feelings of despair. HELP is on the way. Your
attitude and willingness to encounter cancer head on are the
first steps towards finding that help. You guessed it, SELF-
HELP is the beginning point. Trying to help yourself rein-
forces in your own mind that there is hope against cancer.
You need to start by realizing all the assets you have as a
human being to fight and win *any* battle in life's existence.
Those assets are: a sound mind and family love, the power of
your own body's disease fighting immune system, and the
ability to shape attitude with the words from your own
mouth. Give your body a chance to respond to the hope that
your mind and mouth generate through positive thoughts
and words. You must acknowledge and use these potential
weapons if you truly desire to vanquish the threat of cancer.

Choose to fight cancer on *your terms* with positive attitude,
positive speech, positive imaging and God. Do not let cancer
bully you into fighting on its terms of negative attitude,
negative speech, negative imaging and without God. Assert
your attitude from the moment you are confronted with the
mental death sentence that cancer implies. Command upbeat
thoughts, speak confidently, see yourself only in healthy
situations and let God be the overseer of these efforts.

**For God has not given us a spirit of fear, but of
power and of love and of a sound mind.**
2nd TIMOTHY 1:7

After establishing your own positive attitude the next line
of defense is to lean on the support systems available. Foremost, will probably be your spouse or an immediate family
member. For me, my wife, Karen Marie Rockman, was like a
heavy duty shock absorber. She was there to cushion the
bumps and help dodge the pitfalls. Without her I couldn't
have made the trek successfully. Karen's unconditional love,
faith and support were a daily ration of positive attitude. To

her unheralded credit, no matter how bad things got, she could always look past the circumstances and see a rainbow on *our* horizon. Always.

Karen made sacrifice after personal sacrifice with no guaranteed return on her investment of special love. She seldom whimpered and never complained. She spoke and lived *faith* in my eventual outcome before I ever knew what the word meant. Karen and our children instilled me with daily motivation. The sad truth is that at many points of this ordeal it would have been much easier to roll over and die than it was to walk and live. With this truth only a thought away, I tried never to lose sight of the fact that I was battling for more than myself. Much because of my responsibilities as a husband and father I fought to live. If you grasp what cancer can emotionally do to a family you will understand where I'm coming from. Basically, when cancer claims a family member through death it opens the door to allow the disease to hereditarily intimidate the remaining family members. Again, cancer is a monstrous bully.

MAKING MEDICINE WORK FOR YOU

If available, let medicine assist your personal efforts with caring, competent doctors and proper treatment. Confidence and trust in your doctor is a must. The treatment he or she prescribes requires mutual trust between doctor and patient. Even if the prescribed treatment is *no treatment*, it still demands an unwritten contract of faith in the patient/doctor relationship. Trust the medical doctors of your choice without putting the whole burden of your care and cure on their shoulders.

These next few paragraphs are very important if my personal experience with cancer is going to make a contribution towards helping anyone. In order to use the medical world's expertise to your advantage you must understand the role and function of your doctors and the medicine at their disposal. With this perspective, there are three significant areas which need to be addressed in detail. *FIRST*, I encourage you to insist that your doctor be honest in his appraisal of your prognosis and treatment. You have to know what you're facing before you can prepare a defense. Do not accept the diluted truth. There is a drastic need for cancer patients to change their own passive approach to cancer and its treatment. Aggressive, positive attitude needs to become the norm not remain the exception.

From the moment cancer is discovered in your body you should be aware of the seriousness and ready to fight back. I don't mean panicked aware, I mean informed aware. People, both young and old, are dying without a fight. Many of them seem to prefer to take the *Alice in Wonderland* approach, naively believing that their path will end up at its predestined point no matter what route they choose to take. Please understand that at the end of this *"yellow brick road"* you may find a hearse instead of a rainbow.

My frankness is intentional. I am trying to help you save your life and maintain quality of life. Some patients foster this "come what may" attitude on their own, while in other instances their doctors and well-meaning family members unknowingly encourage this naive ignorance. I feel strongly that the cancer victim MUST get involved in his or her own battle. This is a mandatory requirement. If docility is truly your choice of approach then I sincerely wish you good luck. From what I've gone through myself and witnessed with other cancer victims, the disease of cancer is much too aggressive for passive approaches to effectively work.

SECOND, once your doctors have leveled with you to the best of their ability, it's your turn for action. Even if it's a worst case scenario of terminal diagnosis don't give up. Your doctors are human beings, in most instances they are going to draw foregone conclusions based on their own observations and knowledge of cancer. For example: Hypothetically, let's suppose that your doctor is a cancer specialist who has seen 25 people in the past two years with the same type of cancer with which you have just been diagnosed. Out of those 25 persons, one lived and 24 died. It doesn't require an I.Q. of 240 to figure out the probable conclusion of your doctor. You just fell into the terminal category. In your doctor's mind you most likely just entered the world of the living dead. Alive, and here for the moment, but soon-to-be dead and gone.

Remember, their understanding of the situation is based on medical data and statistics, NOT on familiarity with your personality. In most cases, a doctor does not know the patient well enough to realize what weapons the patient has mentally and spiritually brought to the fight against cancer. This is an unknown in your favor. The doctor does not have any idea as to your ability or desire to activate the body's disease fighting neuropeptides. These are neutralizing proteins in each of us that activate or supercharge the human anatomy's immune system. They are antibodies with which we were born. Medicine and your doctor do not have the last say on how your battle will be waged. You do! Use all the weapons you have at your command and start with your own attitude. Think positive and speak positive.

THIRD, treatment needs to be much more aggressive when treating cancer with the goal of defeating the disease. Month after month, I see more and more cancer patients enduring chemotherapy but only prolonging their life. I watch the amounts of chemo drugs being administered to them and have to wonder what the medicine is striving to attain. People lay in their hospital beds and tell me they are handling the chemotherapy just fine. Well, in my opinion, if they are indeed "just fine" then they aren't getting strong enough dosages. Chemo is toxic. Therefore, I have to think that if you put enough toxic drugs into a cancer patient's veins to truly combat malignancy and spreading, that cancer patient will be very sick instead of "just fine." It's time to let the cancer victims determine the concrete aim of their treatment and proceed from there.

Take this to the bank. My goal as I resisted cancer was always complete, uncompromised victory over the disease. Aware of this, I was never "just fine" as I endured chemotherapy. With the heavy doses of chemo and the tight regimen under which they were administered at M.D. Anderson, I was very sick for a long time. The sickness from chemo drugs being infused was something I had accepted as part of my effort to beat cancer and return to quality life and health. If you are truly going to pull out all the stops in battling cancer then give medicine the green light to use aggressive treatment.

Once you've incorporated this three step formula, understand that you are going to have some bad hours and even some bad days along the way. We are human beings, *not* super human beings. Your goal should be to have more good hours and days than bad. That means more days of assertive, positive thinking than other days of negative thoughts and self-pity. Do not riddle yourself with reproach over some bad times. You can doubt in your mind as long as you believe in your heart. Try to at least start each day on a positive note and end each day the same way. This routine can only help you.

One very important conclusion came to me often during the writing of this book. What I was putting down on paper had been lived and felt many times by many people. Nothing I was jotting in my journal at M.D. Anderson was terribly different than the trials and tribulations of other cancer patients who I came in contact with daily. We were enduring cancer and its treatment in the present just as others had endured it in the past and still others would endure it in the future.

The emotions and experiences I was writing about were basically the same for everyone. We all had the best doctors and latest medical technology available. We all had to deal with dark, negative thoughts by utilizing our own defenses. We all had various support systems; usually our spouse or an immediate family member as the primary one. Our personal approach may have varied immensely but our goal was exactly the same. We ALL wanted to rid our body of cancer and our minds of the doubts that accompany the disease. Therefore, what I felt as I faced cancer was not unique; it was only recorded. My prayers to God were not original; they were just admitted. Even my conclusions had been drawn before; they simply had not been stated. Personal observations, experiences and impressions, they add up to potential help for present and future cancer victims. Use the resources you have to *HELP YOURSELF* defeat cancer!

WHERE DOES GOD FIT IN?

God is alive and well. He fits in everywhere if we let him. How do I know this? Because he touched our lives in so many distinct ways. During our six month saga of diagnosis and treatment. Karen and I were seemingly escorted through several areas of potential disaster. These topics have been mentioned in previous chapters as they occurred. I don't think we were able to appreciate the uncommon rarity as much back then as we can now in looking back and realizing, "Wow, were we ever fortunate!" God's guiding hand and gentle touch were subtly evident from onset to finish.

The unusual circumstances stand out in both our minds and merit repeating. First off, we were led from Flint, Michigan to Houston, Texas like a horse drawn to water. Despite wanting the huge tumor surgically removed I wisely opted to see Dr. James Cox for a second opinion. This was uncharacteristic for me. I'm a notorious believer in quick, clean solutions. Immediate surgery at Flint Osteopathic Hospital would have satisfied my definition of a quick and clean removal of the problem. Why didn't I go through with the scheduled surgery? I don't really know. At the time, we followed our instincts instead of my short-sighted wishes. Again, we felt led and actually directed to M.D. Anderson Cancer Clinic. Even back then, Karen and I were certain it was the correct move.

Next, there was the indisputable point that the huge tumor in my abdomen continued to shrink in size despite Dr. Logothetis' opinion that it would probably not shrink anymore. Going back through our journal notes verifies that Logo told us on three different occasions not to count on the tumor shrinking any further. Especially, after it had enlarged following the first chemo treatment. From Logo's reaction and regular appraisal I would have to say the tumor shrinking was at the very least unexpected or out of the medical ordinary. To us, it was excitingly unusual to watch my tumor react different than most and yet in a positive direction. Medical data supported the scarcity of this development.

Also on the list of uncommon events was the reality that my aorta and vena cava never sustained permanent damage from the tumor straddling my spine. It was kind of amazing that the blood supply to my lower limbs was not pinched off by the tumor as it initially grew and infringed on these two large veins which run parallel to the spine. At least three of my friends and fellow patients had been threatened by a similarly located tumor. In each case, their respective aortas or vena cavas had been pinched off until massive swelling occurred in their legs and feet. Along the same lines, my internal organs were threatened from day one by the large size and precarious location of my tumor and yet escaped with no real damage. It seemed highly unusual that I was able to dodge all these potential complications.

Last on the list was the medical fact that no primary site was ever found. They [the doctors] searched high and low for this site which emitted the malignant tumor, so it was certainly not due to an oversight or lack of effort. For the type of cancer which I was treated, this was truly an amazing development. Let's qualify the lack of a primary site by merely stating that with non-seminoma germ cell tumor of the testis this outcome was extremely unusual. Logo and medical statistics attested to the rareness.

NOT A MIRACLE

I think I've made it clear that *I do not* claim to be a medical miracle...just an unusual case. At the same time, I've attempted to concisely offer some not-so-easy to explain circumstances which took place during my treatment. You'll have to draw your own comfortable conclusions. I have.

If you still insist on a bonafide "miracle healing" that is documented by medical doctors, it should be clear that you'll have to look elsewhere. I suggest Dodie Osteen's book *Healed of Cancer* or a man named Harry DeCamp's short booklet, titled *One Man's Miracle*. I've since discovered that there are quite a number of books and stories presenting documented miracles of healing. You simply have to look for them in out of the way places. If you ask the logical question, "Why doesn't the American public hear or read about more miracles?" The answer is [in my opinion] that good news doesn't travel nearly as fast as bad news. Sadder yet, good news doesn't sell as well as bad news. Pick up a daily newspaper or turn on the television set's six o'clock news if you don't believe me. Bad news seems to make sensational news while good news seems to make no news at all.

Now, if you DO NOT insist on a "miracle healing" but DO believe in miracles, then read on. I am NOT a miracle healing in the strict medical sense. For my own self-assurance I don't need to be. Actually, I don't even want to be a recognized miracle healing. The notoriety scares me. On the other hand, no one will ever convince me that a miracle did not happen in my life. You see, I finally have those assurances and guarantees I searched so very long to find. They did not come just from being tough and a fighter. They did not come from medicine. They did not come from diet, vitamins or exercise. They came from believing in the promises of a God I've never seen.

What those assurances and guarantees have given me is a new lease on life. In the last year [September '89 thru September '90], Karen and I have returned to Houston, Texas and M.D. Anderson Cancer Clinic four times. For these quarterly scheduled checkups I am put through all the old tests as my doctors search for cancer one more time. During these examinations, all the old doubts and fears would like to surface. They can't because I refuse to give them a foothold. We go there with peace of mind and return with peace of mind. That peace of mind has been confirmed each time with an *A-OK*, cancer free checkup. I can thank only God for that reassuring feeling of inner peace. Thanks to *His Word*, I believe I am healed forever of cancer. I live each day like I am healed forever. I think, talk and act each day secure in that knowledge. Cancer does not bully me and I firmly believe it never will.

Following this opinionated discussion of God you might be envisioning a halo around my head. Once again, you better look elsewhere. If you require an angel for credibility then you are out of luck because I am certainly no angel. I'm as human as they come. I prove it every day of my life as I encounter impatience, temper, selfishness and a demanding personality within myself. In fact, once in awhile, I still get the urge to come up alongside someone's head when all else fails to gain their sometimes obnoxious attention. Just an urge mind you, but it lends credence to the admission that you'll find no halo around this head. I try to live God's formula for life instead of my own. When applied, it works much better than mine ever did.

If I felt that the reader knew the promises of God which I stumbled onto I would not waste so many words discussing the topic. My audience would probably know more than I could possibly present. Since I don't believe this to be the case, I've taken the liberty to assume that God's healing promises are news to quite a few uninformed cancer victims. Because of that assumption you have been exposed to a considerable amount of references to prayer and this God of ours. Let me share something I learned from that exposure: You are not going to find the inner peace and assurances you need anywhere else — *the God Almighty of the Bible* is the only answer when it comes to defeating the mind-haunting thoughts of spreading, metastasizing and reoccurrence. Medicine comes up short. Diet and vitamins come up short. Exercise and raw sunlight come up short. Depending on just yourself comes up short. God is that "higher authority" for which you are searching. When you truly believe that, cancer will no longer chase you.

Theology is not my field of expertise but I do know that logic and facts cannot explain the concept of God. The image of a God falls into the supernatural realm. I cannot explain what God is all about. I don't have to! God does His own explaining. That's what the big, black covered book probably laying somewhere in your home is for...the Bible explains the concept of God. It is there to know and understand Him on

His terms. It contains what He offers us as human beings and what He expects from us in return. For me, *His Word* ended up being medicine in its purest form.

The God most of us direct our prayers towards just wouldn't be all knowing if He didn't realize mankind's tendency to let fear and insecurity be our often dominating emotions. That's why most of us are afraid to acknowledge his presence and influence in our lives — fear and insecurity. We're embarrassed to worship something we can't see or touch. Let's face it, it's hard to talk to a God we never see and seldom feel. It's almost impossible to trust in Him. Our family, friends and peers might laugh and ridicule.

Then along comes sickness. And that sickness is a deadly disease. The cancer that always seemed to be striking some-one else — a relative, a friend, a celebrity — is now striking you. All of a sudden it doesn't matter who might laugh or ridicule your belief in God because you are fighting for your life. Your back is against the wall and you are searching for a cure to your specific disease. The God dilemma suddenly disappears. The God hang-up is no longer an obstacle. Why? Because when the medical field's expertise offers no remedy and death seems imminent...God is all we have left. In my own mind, I am sure that He would like to see us come to his doorstep and establish a relationship before the chips are down. But, since He is also a merciful God, He seems to unconditionally accept the circumstances that finally send us His way. One of those circumstances is fear. Pure, unadulter-ated fear. In my case terminal cancer fear.

For myself, I don't have to explain or justify the existence of God. I can't see the air we breathe but I know it's there. I can't touch the love I have for my wife and children but I know it's there. Well, God is just as obvious to me. His presence was apparent to Karen and myself in all areas of our cancer ordeal.

After my experience, I'm totally convinced there are a large number of people walking around out there who be-lieve in the same God I do. And the same way. Some are sick right now and some are going to be sick one day in the future. For obvious reasons, they may be hesitant to admit their religious beliefs and brandish their faith more boldly. That also is fine because knowing God is a private, personal and spiritual relationship. But you see, I didn't afford myself that luxury, I made some personal commitments and one of those commitments was to *"...declare the works of the Lord."*

In other words, acknowledge God and give him credit for guiding me through a cancerous situation which I could not control. Maybe my opinion on God's contribution seems far fetched, after all it's only an opinion. You will have to judge for yourself. At the risk of being labeled a bible thumper, I honestly feel that the peace that came to me as I fought cancer is an *understatement* of our unseen God's contribution. Controversy never bothered me before so I am sure not going to let it start bothering me now. As a whole, I've always felt that people love to gossip. Perhaps this little three letter word called *God* will give them something to talk about. If it does, that's a start in the right direction to beating cancer or any other life threatening disease.

REINFORCED CONCLUSIONS

My own observations at M.D. Anderson Cancer Clinic and impressions at home have since been reinforced. They have also lead me to some candid views. Without mincing words, many cancer victims DO NOT get involved enough in their own fight. Most cancer victims DO NOT realize it is a three stage battle which involves defeating cancer emotionally, physically and financially. And in that order. Many cancer victims DO NOT want to carry the burden of their own cure. They unconsciously want the doctor and medicine to fight their battle. Finally, many cancer victims DO NOT consider God as a legitimate source for conquering fear and bodily healing. They ignore the potential of God as our creator.

Mankind builds things with the idea in mind that if it breaks it can be fixed. Well, I believe that God designed the human anatomy the same way. *He* holds the patent and must be able to help fix something *He* himself designed and created. If you are going to resist cancer successfully then use every asset within your means — and that includes God. The very first asset is yourself and your own mental attitude and preparation. Don't settle for less than your best daily effort — and take one day at a time.

The message I am offering is not based on what I personally accomplished. It is based solely on what I learned and perceived to do *different*. I have never undersold my mental and physical toughness throughout the whole ordeal. I have never underestimated the importance of my wife and family's love. I have never undermined the value of competent medicine under the supervision of caring doctors. But, let's set the record straight. I can give you the names of twenty-five different people who were tough, had supportive love and the best medicine money could afford. They are all dead. When mankind's medicine came up short they may have overlooked one possible element in their search for help against cancer. They possibly overlooked a God who represented the only hope they had when the final analysis came in. Only they will ever know for sure.

These impressions led me to the lonely conclusion that my personal efforts were never going to satisfy the need for guarantees and assurances. *Faith was the difference.* It was the difference in handling cancer or allowing it to bully me on every front. It was the difference in possessing a lifetime of peaceful assurances or allowing the domination of agonizing fear. It was the difference which many times separated the living from the dead.

In closing, two overriding thoughts helped me cope with cancer on a daily basis. Both of these conclusive thoughts were arrived at the hard way... through trial and error. I'd like to share them in the hope they help someone else. First of all, the hospital environment in which Karen and I were trapped, continually echoed an unmistakable message about the world in which we live. *"Life is neither fair nor easy, it's how you handle it that counts."* In other words, the world we live in is full of grief. You can go around frowning and living the *"Poor Me's"* or you can smile and live the *"I'm OK's."* The choice is yours.

Secondly, as human beings we are products of our own tongue. We are what we say and we live what we speak. Another way of expressing this philosophy is, *"Positive words promote positive results and negative words promote negative results."* Again, the choice is yours.

These simple thoughts helped keep my attitude in perspective each day. They amount to acknowledging the grief of reality and yet looking past it to a better day ahead. Regardless of circumstances try to think positive and speak positive. Mental imagery and busy exercise promote good attitude. Picture yourself in ONLY healthy situations from the past; for the present; and in the future.

The bottom line is that God does indeed fit into all aspects of cancer. Before your personal cancer battle is over you will need the assurances of that higher authority. Between complications, spreading and reoccurrence, cancer will chase you like a bogeyman and lurk around every corner. Especially if medicine draws the line at your type of cancer and God is the ONLY hope you have left.

I wrote for a single purpose. That purpose was to offer a chance at the same peace of mind which I found to defeat cancer. I've confided my fears. I've told you of my doubts. I've shared my skepticism. What's left? Just the victory over all these and more. For me, the victory is in the commitment of the words I have come to believe and understand:

...with God all things are possible.
Matthew 19:26

In the final analysis, I have said many things about the disease of cancer and touched many areas associated with cancer. With an interrogative format I would like to state some of my formed opinions one last time: Have I guaranteed the shrinking and disappearance of your specific tumor? *No, I haven't.* Have I promised you remission for your type of leukemia? *No, I haven't.* Have I assured you that your cancer will not metastasize? *No, I haven't.* Have I declared immunity to reoccurrence? *No, I haven't.* Finally, have I offered you false hope. *No, I certainly haven't.* But, I HAVE GIVEN YOU THE PATH TO TRUE PEACE OF MIND. The healing scriptures contained in the Bible are the medicine at the end of that path. They are more than a tourniquet to stop the bleeding. They are a transfusion of faith that renders genuine peace of mind. That is what it takes to beat cancer or any other terminal disease...peace of mind...inner peace. Why do I say this? Because you must confront cancer emotionally before you can ever truly beat it physically. It's a personal battle that begins in the realm of your own mind and finishes in your heart.

I cannot guarantee that you will defeat cancer and live a long, prosperous life. That is personal, between you, God and medicine. I can guarantee that sincere belief in *God's word*, not mine, will give you the inner peace it takes to handle anything which comes your way. That includes cancer and all its ugly details. I BEAT CANCER. With God as the overseer, the love and support of your family and good doctors...YOU CAN TOO! Because when hope in the final outcome becomes faith in a higher authority you are there. Cancer no longer can chase you into mental submission. Remember, you treat cancer with medicine but you beat cancer with God.

Chapter 11

THE EPILOGUE

After learning to handle the fear that comes with cancer I feel safe in the sentiment that I can handle any setbacks life sends my way. With Karen at my side, I overcame the fear and God gave the assurances. Looking back, we were quite a team. At this point in time, sixteen months after surgery and twenty-two months since the discovery of the malignant tumor in my abdomen, we have recovered as a family from the curse of cancer. Karen is back doing what she loves and does best; functioning as a full-time mom and housewife. The kids schedules keep her jumping but she enjoys being involved. She works in bowling and shopping for her leisure time excursions. Not necessarily in that order. Though cancer exacted its toll emotionally, Karen finds daily comfort knowing our cancer episode is finally in her past.

All of our kids are back on track and growing up much too fast. Melissa, our oldest, is now graduated from high school and enrolled as a full-time student in a travel agent program. She aspires to get into flight attendant school with a major airlines when she reaches the minimum age requirement. The travel agent program supposedly affords an inside track. Cheryl is our second oldest child. She is a senior in high school and is talking about going to college to be an elementary level school teacher. The biggest thing in her life at this moment is boys and preparing for "the real world." She plans to run track in the Spring after lettering last year.

Next in line is our oldest son, Ricky. He's a high school sophomore. He loves football and riding his motorcycle dirt bike. The neighbors don't seem to care for his loud motorcycle nearly as much as he does. He plans on college but girls and a part-time job occupy his priorities right now. Then comes Stacey, our twelve year old who is going on eighteen. She thinks so anyway. Stacey is in the middle school and has graduated to a "big kid" status since she now rides the bus with all the older kids. Her most recent claim to fame is that she has more telephone conversations in a day than most of us have in a month. Randy, our ten year old, is last in the line. Randy loves sports and is a fifth grader in the elementary school. Twelve months a year he's busy in one sport or another. Since he's the youngest, Randy qualifies as his mom's "baby." He keeps Karen busy just buying shoes for him as he wears them out in record setting time.

It goes without saying that my wife and I count our blessings each and every day. Even though we've been home for over a year neither of us ever completely forget our recent past which included a cancer induced time of separation from our children. The Houston experience helps us appreciate that even the "bad days" of hectic, everyday living are really good ones. Our family is intact and healthy. Love, in the form of discipline and supervision, are constant reminders to our brood that mom and dad are home for good. And that's after the real love of praise and affection. Despite some of their adolescent complaints the kids are secure once again in our presence.

Brings us down to me. Emotionally, cancer left a lot of painful memories but no permanent scars. I learned much from the experience and never dwell in the past on what might have been. The more cancer victims I come in contact with the more I consider myself one of a fortunate few. I continue to take one day at a time.

Financially, it has been an uphill struggle. As the head of the household and designated breadwinner it's been difficult to accept that all our resources have been drained by my cancer. The bills keep coming while the money long ago ran out. Before cancer struck I thought we were well-prepared for a rainy day. We had savings accounts, retirement insurance policies, college funds for the kids and even some precious metals and stocks. It wasn't enough. Cancer ended up being much more than a "rainy day." As I alluded to throughout this book, life in the cancer lane is a three stage battle. After defeating cancer emotionally and physically, our financial woes are the final stage of the dark journey. I'm not crying and my family is not starving but those are the hard financial facts. We've had a lot of help from family and friends and will be back on our feet in the near future. God willing, that's a promise now and soon to be a fact.

Physically, my body still has some lingering effects from chemotherapy. My short term memory continues to be a problem. I don't seem to remember details one minute after they are said. If I don't write things down as they happen I soon forget. It has literally been a matter of *out of sight, out of mind*. I'm aware it's a problem area and work on it often throughout a day with little memory exercises. The numbness which struck during my third course of chemo remains. My left leg, arm and hand still go numb and ache occasionally. When I jog [maybe I should say try to jog] or drive a car especially. I still have some of those bruise marks on my arms and feet which mysteriously appeared during my fourth chemo session. Some have disappeared, hopefully the rest will fade with time. Then there is my hearing which is definitely damaged. I seem to have a considerable loss of hearing in my left ear and inability to filter out background noise in both ears. I spend a lot of time asking "Huh?" and "What?"

I seldom say much about these chemo holdovers. The problems sound worse than they actually are. I feel they are gradually getting better. In my own mind, I know they'll go away — just don't know when. Day to day, I try to practice what I preach and maintain a positive attitude. It helps to remind myself that some of my old friends and fellow patients would love to be alive and experiencing any of these latent side effects. That kind of says it all, don't you think?

LAST PATIENT UPDATE
THROUGH DECEMBER 1990
In spite of the fact that I deplore cancer statistics because

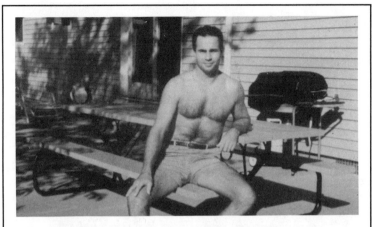

The "better days" I'd anticipated were here. I felt great!

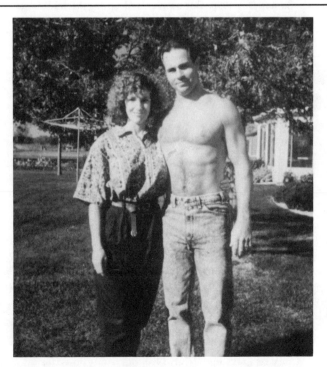

Labor Day weekend 1990. What a difference a year makes!

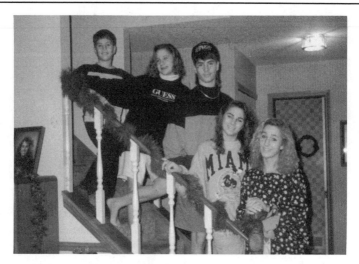

Christmas Day 1990. Our brood lined up for the traditional stairway shot before raiding their presents.

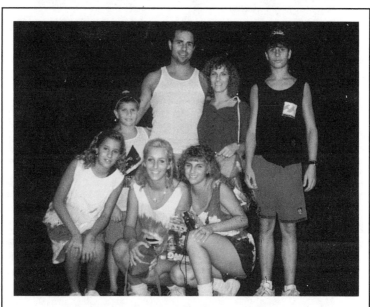

One year after surgery (July 1990), our family posed for an impromptu photo at Disneyworld in Orlando, Fla.

they diminish the human element, I feel compelled to make you aware of the latest data available. According to the Sloan-Kettering Cancer Research Center, over 490,000 Americans died in 1989 of this disease. Probably more discouraging is the fact that cancer still strikes two out of every three American families. In 1990 the projected death toll will easily surpass the half million mark. I present these facts for one reason: cancer is not going to just fade away. It appears that this 20th century affliction is here to stay so we better figure out how to fight this tenacious disease — and win. Following are the names of some who have already fought their battle. These cancer patients were human beings long before they were ever considered medical statistics. Rightfully so, they also have a final cancer story to tell.

Let's begin with Kevin "M", who as of this date, is back home in Corpus Christi, Texas. Kevin, his wife, Tina and their two-year old daughter, Carrie are doing as well as can be expected. For what Kevin went through I think he's doing terrific. He is back to work although he still suffers effects from that last dose of chemotherapy administered in May of '89. His feet continue to give him pain and discomfort but Kevin is a tough customer and I feel sure that eventually this complication will disappear. Like me, his hearing and memory are more than a little suspect. Hopefully, these areas will improve. Positive attitude and time are in his favor. We try to talk by phone every couple of months and remain close friends with future plans of getting together with each other and our families.

Dwight "P" and Carl "M" succumbed to the ravages of cancer in early 1990. We discovered through the patient grapevine that Carl died at home, back in Missouri. He was another cancer story which dragged on for almost two years. If you haven't been there you can't begin to comprehend what it is to fight for your life over an extended period of time. Imagine two years amidst the constant turmoil of cancer playing on your emotions. For his own peace of mind, we hope Carl spent some meaningful time while at home before he passed away. Dwight is finally out of pain. His cancer struggle had been one that included many complications and much pain. I'll miss him and the serious conversations we shared. His wife, Elizabeth, was a beautiful person and tremendous support system. Karen and I offer our deepest sympathy to Elizabeth and their adult children.

Peter "G" and Eddie "T" are doing fine by all accounts. Peter went through Hell during his treatment. Complications and side effects were a never ending diversion that seemed to stalk his chemotherapy and radiation courses. Peter is finally back to work and trying to pick up his young life where cancer left it off. His impaired vision [due to a metastatic brain tumor] continues to be an obstacle he will have to deal with the rest of his life. But, he is alive and could be much worse off. Eddie "T" is alive as far as we know. I haven't seen or heard from Eddie since the day he walked out of M.D. Anderson to go home before his body was actually ready. If you recall, he'd just received his last course of Cisca II with cisplatin. We assume he is alive because he would have to be treated at M.D. Anderson if problems arose. They have no current information on him. Leaning on the old adage that "No news is good news;" we think and hope the best for Eddie.

Vince "M" and Pat "M" are both gone now. Vince died in April 1990 at M.D. Anderson while we were there for my six month checkup. In the last two months which Karen and I spent at M.D. Anderson we became good friends with Vince and his wife, Gloria. I still remember them taking me out to dinner just prior to my surgery in July of '89. They felt sorry for me because I was alone for the few days Karen had remained in Michigan with our children. We had a lot of fun that evening. Cancer stole another good human being when it claimed Vince. Gloria has since set up a cancer memorial fund in honor of Vince back in their home state of New Jersey. Pat succumbed to cancer in September of 1990. He had recently married his longtime fiance, Judy. Ironically, his death occurred on the day that Karen and I flew into Houston for my one year checkup. Pat's death hit close to home. We had visited with Pat and Judy quite often following my surgery. They were warm and friendly company. Like almost every couple we encountered at M.D. Anderson Cancer Clinic they were a team in their battle against cancer. Pat has finally found peace and escaped the fear which cancer bred. We'll miss him.

Phil "C" is still fighting his metastasized cancer. He is doing as well as he possibly can. Karen and I bumped into him during my one year checkup as we awaited my turn for a C.A.T. scan. He looked good physically and spoke very positive. We both enjoyed talking to him and sent our greetings to his wife, Marjorie Ann. She had stayed behind in Florida to look after their affairs while Phil made the trip to M.D. Anderson for comparison tests on his tumor. Although he admits to getting tired easily, Phil is working full time and battling his cancer just as full time. He is not only a good person and caring human being, he is also one very strong individual. At this point, Phil is once again scheduled for future surgery and currently is taking experimental drugs within the chemotherapy program. He has been and will remain in our prayers.

"Crazy Mel" never did get back to see me. I spotted him one time following our wild conversation in the hospital parking lot, and this quick glance was from a distance as I walked the concourse bordering the front of M.D. Anderson. Tried to flag him down at that time but he could not hear my voice over the cars zooming past. He didn't look well that day but I'm not going to pronounce his death sentence. It takes all kinds of different personalities to make up this world and Mel was most assuredly a "different personality." In a way, Mel was a breath of fresh air. Nothing seemed to get him down. Even though I felt his blase attitude towards cancer was superficial it apparently worked for him. I seldom argue with results. You can be sure of one thing, wherever Mel is it will not be boring!

A happy ending which has not been mentioned previously is a giant of a young man named David "D" from Texas. I met him near the end of my treatment. He was just over six feet tall and weighed 265 pounds the day he came into M.D. Anderson Cancer Clinic for treatment. The bulk was mostly muscle and he looked like man-mountain. When he left M.D. Anderson, after five doses of chemotherapy, he was considerably smaller in stature but cancer free. We got to be pretty good friends in a short amount of time. David was a football player who was playing on a scholarship at a small college in Missouri. Logo and his assistant, Betsy, informed us that David is doing great. His last checkup was a "thumbs up" and he hopes to play football next year. We hope he maintains his present prognosis and continues to do great.

The last patient on our list is one very dear to Karen and myself; my brother Craig. He is doing excellent. As of December 1990, it has been two years since the discovery of his cancer. Craig is now self-employed and working hard at getting his new business established. His wife, Beth, is a certified aerobics instructor. They have a daughter at home who is in the 11th grade and a son going to college at Michigan State University. Craig and Beth are enjoying daily that cancer is a part of their past. Once a year Craig has a detailed checkup at U of M Ann Arbor Hospital in Michigan. Knowing his aversion for doctors and hospitals, I think even this yearly exam may be too often to suit him.

For the Jameses, the Patricks, the Kevins, the Dwights, the Hollys, the Victors, the Johns, the Larrys, the Peters, the Dennises, the Mels, the Elizabeths, the Scotts, the Carls, the Ruths, the Kens, the Jims, the Vinces, the Sids, the Waynes, the Cecils, the Georges, the Elaines, the Eddies, the Bills: For all of these and many more names which represent real people stricken with cancer, the writing of this book was accomplished with your contribution. Your struggle did not go unrecognized. By sharing a glimpse of your daily battle you will never be just statistics to me or my wife. At your expense much of our insight into the world of sickness and disease was acquired. Your reactions and responses to cancer taught us something about ourselves and about human beings in general. You are the main reason I chose to share my story and let it be *our story* of cancer. Each of you lived your own personal cancer story. The living epitaph contained on these pages should reflect that your battle was not in vain.

* * * * * * *

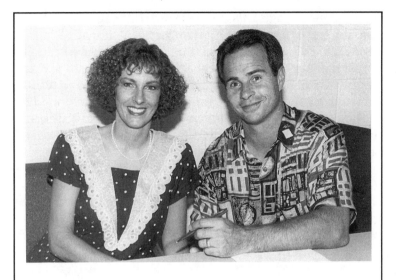

FROM THE AUTHOR(S): Karen and I would like to leave you with one last impression — that of health; an appreciation for each and every day; and an undying faith in the unseen God of the Bible.

Acknowledgements

To my wife, Karen Marie, for tolerating my nightly endeavors to write and finish this book for well over six months of our lives. Thanks for excusing my absence from our bedroom those many nights and just plain putting up with me.

Special and sincere appreciation goes out to two amateur editors who aided my writing efforts with computer programming, cover design and constructive criticism. To my sister, Deborah Rockman and my brother-in-law, Dean Ouellette — I can only say "thank you." Your assistance was immeasurable.

Also, a word of thanks is extended to Dr. William Bischoff. Bill reminded me early in my writing that if I was going to have any chance to help someone else I had to be open and honest with my innermost feelings. It was sound advice and came from a source who "walked a mile in my shoes." Bill courageously waged his own personal fight against terminal disease.

Not to be forgotten at this point, Karen and I would like to extend our heartfelt "thanks" once more to the many people who touched our lives with care and kindness throughout the whole ordeal. We could not have made it without your love and concern. A special thanks goes out to the M.D. Anderson Cancer Center's doctors, nurses and support staff.

To our family and friends, we send our warmest thanks. Your efforts maintained our household and kept our five children safe for our return. Words cannot describe our gratitude. To the groups, organizations and many different church congregations — "thank you" for all the prayers. There is no denying that God was aware of our plight and knew us by name. There is also no denying he answered both your prayers and ours.

Finally, the wives of my fellow patients deserve special recognition for their tour of volunteer duty which they put in at M.D. Anderson. They were and are real "stayers." When things got tough these ladies did not retreat or run, they settled in next to their husbands and stayed for the duration. One more time I will say it, their love and support was irreplaceable. They were quiet and constant companions. In the long run, they were a hidden asset which helped balance the books.

* * * * * * *

1994 REVISION UPDATE:

Phil "C" lost his battle to metastasized cancer in 1991.

Dr. William Bischoff succumbed to amyotrophic lateral sclerosis [Lou Gehrig's disease] in 1992.

As well as being true friends who will be greatly missed, both of these men made considerable contributions to my book writing endeavor. I trust that heaven is now their home and resting place.

My brother Craig received a thumbs up A-OK in January of 1994. He's a thankful cancer survivor who is currently the busy and successful operator of three different businesses.

As for me, my five year check-up in April of 1994 went as

expected; all clear, not a trace of cancer existed anywhere in my body. I thank God for my continued health and peace of mind.

Statisitically, cancer will claim over 538,00 lives in 1994. This means about 1,400 people a day will die of cancer. Over 1.2 million new cases will be diagnosed; and this does not include skin cancers. At present, one out of every five deaths in the United States is from cancer. These statistics supplied by the American Cancer Society [Cancer Facts & Figures - 1994].

* * * * * * *

Rainbow Man

Richard G. Rockman, Jr.